C000150307

Sleep Right, Sleep Tight

Also by Tweddle Child + Family Health Service:

Eat Right, Don't Fight:
A practical guide to feeding children from birth to the preschool years

Sleep Right, Sleep Tight

A practical, proven guide to solving your baby's sleep problems

Tweddle Child + Family Health Service

DOUBLEDAY

SYDNEY • AUCKLAND • TORONTO • NEW YORK • LONDON

SLEEP RIGHT, SLEEP TIGHT
A DOUBLEDAY BOOK

First published in Australia and New Zealand in 2000 by Doubleday
This revised and updated edition first published in 2006
Copyright © Tweddle Child + Family Health Service, 2006

All rights reserved. No part of this publication may be reproduced, stored in a retrieval system,
transmitted in any form or by any means, electronic, mechanical, photocopying, recording or
otherwise, without the prior written permission of the publisher.

National Library of Australia
Cataloguing-in-Publication Entry

Tweddle Child + Family Health Service.
Sleep right, sleep tight.

Rev and updated ed.

ISBN 1 86471 096 9.
ISBN 978 1 86471 096 0.

1. Children – Sleep. 2. Sleep – Health aspects. 3. Sleep
disorders in children – Popular works.
I. Title.

649.122

Transworld Publishers,
a division of Random House Australia Pty Ltd
Level 3, 100 Pacific Highway, North Sydney, NSW 2060
http://www.randomhouse.com.au

Random House New Zealand Limited
18 Poland Road, Glenfield, Auckland

Transworld Publishers,
a division of The Random House Group Ltd
61–63 Uxbridge Road, Ealing, London W5 5SA

Random House Inc
1745 Broadway, New York, New York 10036

Text design by Seymour Designs
Typeset by Midland Typesetters, Australia
Printed and bound by Griffin Press, South Australia

10 9 8 7 6 5 4 3 2

This book is dedicated to all the parents and children who have inspired and supported us in our work at Tweddle. A special thank you to all the parents that wrote in with their thanks and stories of their continued success at home. Your stories have enriched this book. Names have been altered to protect the identity of individuals.

Contents

Acknowledgements	viii
Foreword	ix
Introduction	xi
Chapter 1: Being a parent	1
Chapter 2: About sleep	5
Chapter 3: Babies up to 3 months	19
Chapter 4: Babies 3–6 months old	51
Chapter 5: Babies 6–12 months old	87
Chapter 6: Children 1–4 years old	127
Chapter 7: Multiple births	167
About Tweddle Child + Family Health Service	171
List of resources	173

Acknowledgements

Tweddle Child + Family Health Service wishes to acknowledge the dedication, commitment and professional standards of Tweddle staff in developing and refining the sleep and management strategies outlined in this book.

Tweddle particularly acknowledges and wishes to give credit to previous authors Rosey Cummings, Le Ann Williams and Karen Houghton who were instrumental in developing the book and without whom this new edition would not be possible.

This edition was updated by the current staff at Tweddle. The technical editors were Cate Teague, Le Ann Williams, Ann Hindell and Hazel Spiers.

Foreword

The second edition of *Sleep Right, Sleep Tight* is very welcome and builds very well on the sound theory and practice that thousands of parents have used to meet their family needs since the first edition was released in 1998.

Sleep problems of infants and young children remain among the most common and distressing of problem behaviours reported by parents. Few things have more potential to undermine parenting confidence than a crying and fussing infant who is impossible to settle, or a toddler who simply will not go to bed or who wakes numerous times during the night. Sleep difficulties result in tired, irritable infants and sleep-deprived, tense parents; this combination guarantees a household where nothing goes smoothly and everybody seems on edge all the time.

While some infants seem to settle very quickly into predictable and consistent sleep patterns, others have more difficulty. In many instances, parents trying their best to help the child settle into a routine, inadvertently seem to make things worse. They seek advice from health professionals, from books, and from well-meaning relatives. They try a number of different strategies, sometimes switching quickly from one to the other, in their efforts to help the child achieve a good night's sleep.

As paediatricians, we often see these young children and their parents when there have been sometimes many months of sleep difficulties and when parents, having tried all sorts of different things, are rapidly losing confidence that their child will ever be able to sleep through the night.

Settling an infant or getting a toddler to sleep through the night is not rocket science. There are time-honoured techniques which, if implemented with confidence and consistency, will almost always be successful. *Sleep Right, Sleep Tight* is a proven 'practical guide to solving your baby's sleep problems'. It is based on the methods used successfully at Tweddle Child + Family Health Service for many years. *Sleep Right,*

Sleep Tight is written in the form of a manual, with practical and concrete steps for parents to follow. It has just enough theory to provide the context for the recommendations, but not so much that parents get overwhelmed.

Because the genesis and management of sleep difficulties varies in children of different ages, *Sleep Right, Sleep Tight* provides different sections on babies for different stages of development. It is not the sort of book that parents will read and then put back on the shelf. Instead it is designed to be constantly referred to, written in, and otherwise personalised. I particularly like the Frequently Asked Questions at the end of each chapter. Often parents may read a section in a parenting book, carry out the recommendations and, if they do not work, blame themselves. The Frequently Asked Questions sections give common questions and answers and address the reasons why strategies some-time do not appear to work.

It is also pleasing to see the new chapter that talks to parents about what is 'normal' or 'usual' behaviour in new or young babies and what, as parents, we can expect in those important first weeks and months. So often expectations can be unrealistic and this new chapter gives great tips on learning about your new family and, importantly, enjoying this very short time in a child's life.

Sleep Right, Sleep Tight is an excellent resource, which will be valuable for parents and for those professionals who work with young children experiencing sleep difficulties and their families. It is the culmination of many years of experience of successfully helping these youngsters and their families, and it is pleasing that Tweddle is now sharing this accumulated wisdom with the wider community.

PROFESSOR FRANK OBERKLAID
DIRECTOR, CENTRE FOR COMMUNITY CHILD HEALTH
ROYAL CHILDREN'S HOSPITAL
MELBOURNE

Introduction

Welcome to the second edition of *Sleep Right, Sleep Tight*. The positive feedback we've received from parents has told us that the book has been very valuable in guiding them to achieve more sleep for everyone. In this revised and updated edition we have included new chapters on parenthood and the younger baby as well as reviewing all information and techniques to ensure that they are still valid for parents.

This book has been designed to help you and your child resolve the issues related to settling and sleeping, including achieving longer day sleeps and solid night sleeps. It provides practical, proven advice, suggestions and strategies for helping children to settle and resettle to sleep by themselves. It will also help you to understand the sleep patterns of children, and the importance of sleep for their healthy development.

Begin by reading chapters 1, Becoming a parent, and 2, About sleep. It is especially important to read Chapter 2, which explains the nature and significance of sleep and why sleep difficulties can develop, before putting any of the techniques from the book into practice.

Then move on to the chapter that relates to your child's age. In each chapter, specific techniques for settling and sleep are recommended and explained for that age group. Note that some information is repeated from chapter to chapter as certain principles remain the same regardless of a child's age.

At the end of each chapter you will find charts which you can fill out. By monitoring your progress in this way, any improvement in your child's settling and sleep patterns will become clear.

Settling and sleep problems affect boys and girls equally, but for ease of writing we have used 'she' and 'her' (not he/she) to describe all babies and toddlers. There has also been a lot of discussion about the terms used to describe babies, toddlers and children. There are many ways of defining this. When one mother was asked about this, she said that she still calls her teenagers her babies! The general consensus seems to be that a baby is a baby up to the age of one and then she becomes a toddler or young child. If you call your baby or young child something different from the terms that we have used, substitute the word you prefer when you are reading.

Use this book when you are determined to change your child's and household's inadequate sleep situation. Changing things is not always easy so we have included tips and strategies that will help you stay on track and feel positive about the progress you are making.

All babies and young children are individuals but the techniques and strategies discussed here have been shown to be successful for many families over a long period of time. If your baby or young child has special needs, you may like to talk to your maternal and child health or community health nurse or doctor about what you would like to do to alter your child's sleeping difficulties and how you could adapt our techniques to achieve this.

Rachel [aged 12 months] is now sleeping for a full 12 hours every night. It has made such a difference to our lives. And to all the families who are trying to sort out their lives: persist. It does work. It might be difficult at first but it does work. **SUE**

CHAPTER 1

Being a parent

Parenting through the generations   3

Becoming a parent   4

Welcome to the world of parenting – it is an exciting and ever challenging world as you watch your baby develop into a toddler, pre-schooler, school child, teenager and then an adult. Throughout each of these life stages, together you are learning new things about each other. The changes vary – sometimes subtle, sometimes dramatic – and as a parent you are constantly learning and adapting to the changing needs of your child and family. Then, just when you think that you have mastered one change, another exciting challenge comes along!

Parenting through the generations

A new baby can rejuvenate and bring joy to a family, whether long awaited, planned or as a surprise. The smallness, the look, the sounds, the smell, attract her family to her and her to them. Her presence can be so powerful, it can stir the feelings and memories across the generations from the great grandmother who swears she has her son's nose to the uncle who suddenly finds himself visiting much more frequently. All are keen to be part of this baby's life in various ways, whether it be by repeating their own experiences, passing down family stories, playing and having fun, or assisting in practical everyday tasks. This is how a baby learns to belong. And it is from the memories of our own childhoods in this family that we learn about trusting our intuition of parenting.

A baby's presence can, however, equally create confusion between those generations who may have parented at a different time, in a different way or in a different country. It is often said that life was simple back when kids could play in the street, when one was advised: 'Spare the rod, spoil the child' and 'a woman's place was in the home', leaving the impression that one generation is yearning for times gone by and the next generation feeling left out.

Through the generations we have seen many differences and also inconsistencies about the way to parent. What worked for our parents may not work for us. Many other outside factors also influence the way we parent, such as an increase in the number of mothers returning to paid employment and consequently juggling more commitments. Fewer parents have an extended family to rely on for support and there is a much broader range of family circumstances than ever before.

Along your journey, you will most likely read books offering advice from differing childcare experts as well as receive well-meant advice from friends, family members or perhaps people you have only just met. It is important that you feel comfortable in accepting or declining the advice provided. A simple way to work out whether the advice is useful is to ask yourself the following questions. Does the advice:

◎ Help me keep my baby safe?
◎ Fit within my family life?
◎ Help me enjoy my baby?

And:

◎ Can I see myself using the advice or strategies?

Remember that each baby is unique and by watching and listening to your baby and responding to her needs you will get to know your baby better than anyone else. You will become the expert on your baby.

Becoming a parent

Children's settling and sleep difficulties can cause challenges for some families. These can include stress and conflict for sleep-deprived and exhausted parents and feeding and behavioural changes for young children. Frustrating drawn out bedtime behaviour, short or no daytime sleeps and frequent night time waking can at times make it hard to enjoy your young child. If this is your experience, let us reassure you that you are not alone.

It is important, too, to be aware of what is considered 'normal' behaviour for a baby at different ages as their needs change as they grow. For example, it is considered normal for a young baby to wake 5–7 times overnight.

Parenting can be challenging and difficult and what will be a problem for one family may not be a problem for another family. We may cope differently in various situations depending on what else is happening in our lives. Our cultural background, the way we were brought up, society's expectations of parents and our own perceptions and beliefs about parenting are just some of the factors that influence how we respond. What is important is that you do what feels right for you and your family, have realistic expectations and set realistic goals.

At any time if you are concerned about your baby or child's health, we encourage you to see your child health nurse and/or local doctor.

CHAPTER 2

About sleep

Parents' tiredness	7
Getting started	7
Myths about sleep	9
What is a sleeping problem?	9
Why are some children wakeful?	10
The aim of the settling and sleep techniques	12
Understanding sleep	13
How do we sleep?	13
Sleep messages	15
Sleep associations	15
Sleep for babies and young children	16
Personal notes	18

CHARTS

Feed, play, sleep chart	17

Parents' tiredness

Being a parent is exciting, fulfilling and challenging. However, parenting can also be extremely tiring, especially when your young child has a settling or sleep problem. Parents can end up feeling not only tired, but tense, impatient and frustrated from lack of sleep. Often in this situation it is difficult for parents to support each other and relationships may suffer. If you are a sole parent, the responsibility of parenthood may seem overwhelming when compounded by lack of sleep. And parents' sleep deprivation, coupled with a child's grizzly sleep-deprived behaviour, may reduce the enjoyment of the new baby.

Other children in the family may also feel the effects of sleep deprivation, either directly through lack of sleep or indirectly through the effects of having constantly tired and irritable parents.

Getting started

Before you begin to read about sleep and implement the techniques suggested, it may be helpful to stop and consider how your present situation is making you feel. Write it down. In fact, use the following space to make some simple notes.

How do you feel now and what do you want to do?

Before starting on this program it is important to identify what you want to achieve. Write your goals down so that you don't forget the big picture in the wee small hours of a dark night when your baby is unsettled and crying. Clearly stating your goals and keeping them easily accessible will help you achieve what you are seeking.

For example, if bedtime in your house has become a battleground you might like to write: 'By the end of next week we will have had two nights when my baby went to her bed calmly'. You may actually want a better result than this but it is helpful to set an attainable goal. Then you will be pleasantly surprised when you and your baby exceed your goals!

My/our goals for our family's settling and sleep program are:

GOAL 1:

GOAL 2:

GOAL 3:

At the end of each chapter are charts that you can use to track your progress. When filled out over successive nights, these will provide you with evidence of your baby or child's improvement in sleeping patterns and the decreasing amounts of time that you need to spend settling your child. There are also suggestions for management plans to help you work out in advance what you will do during the day or night, such as who is going to be involved in the settling, who is going to look after your other children, and so on.

> Harry [aged 18 months] now sleeps in his cot for 11 hours a night and 2 hours during the day. He is a much happier little boy. I'm sure this is because he feels so good now that he is getting the proper amount of sleep. **WENDY**

Many parents find it difficult to implement a settling and sleep program and benefit from the discussion and assistance of a support person who has also read this book. Do not hesitate to ask for the help and support of a trusted friend or relative. Remember that many families experience similar problems to your own and so do not be afraid or embarrassed to ask for help.

It is important to believe in yourself as a parent as you set about changing your child's settling and sleep patterns. Be assured that the techniques outlined in this book are based on extensive and successful practice. Many parents have already used these strategies to establish better sleeping habits for their children. The rewards will be enormous for you, for your child and for the whole family.

Myths about sleep

MYTH 1:
All babies and toddlers sleep as much as they need.
FALSE: Some babies and toddlers may become more active with tiredness and therefore do not know when they need sleep.

MYTH 2:
Babies and toddlers will grow out of their catnaps and/or night waking. It is just a stage they are going through.
FALSE: Babies and toddlers need sleep. There are phases in a baby's development that will cause them to wake. A continued inability to settle and sleep, however, is not a normal stage of development and assistance may be required to help young children learn to self settle and sleep well.

MYTH 3:
Babies and toddlers don't have sleeping problems.
FALSE: Sleeping problems in young children are common and result in feelings of distress and exhaustion for many parents, and overtired, grizzly children.

What is a sleeping problem?

Families are all different. What is a problem for some people will not be a problem for others. Often, however, poor sleep patterns are established before parents realise what has happened. They then feel unsure how to alter them.

Individuals have varying sleep patterns and sleep needs. Generally for babies and toddlers a sleep problem can be said to exist when one or more of the following continues to occur:

◎ Frequent waking, yet your child is not hungry or thirsty.
◎ Sleeping for short periods only (less than one hour), commonly referred to as 'catnapping'.
◎ The need to be rocked, fed or cuddled in order to fall asleep.
◎ Settling to sleep late at night and then waking early in the morning.

> Grant [my partner] and I are now best friends. For the last few months we have hardly been able to say anything nice to each other because we were both so tired. Even our friends and family are amazed at the changes in us. **DEBBIE**

Sleeping problems are said to affect 15–35 per cent of babies, toddlers and their families. If settling or sleep is a problem with your baby or toddler it does not mean you are a 'failure' or a 'bad' parent.

Trust and believe in yourself and, by using the knowledge and techniques developed with families at Tweddle over very many years, you will learn how to change your situation.

Why are some children wakeful?

There are many reasons why some children either do not settle themselves to sleep or wake before they have had enough sleep during the day or night. The most common reasons are:

- ◎ When a young child is overtired, going to sleep and staying asleep can be difficult.
- ◎ If there are no set patterns in a child's day there are no cues to tell the child when it is sleep time.
- ◎ Changes within the family, such as moving from a cot to a bed, a different room, a new house, going on holidays and starting childcare can contribute to a sleep difficulty.
- ◎ Parents' confusion about what signs indicate a baby or child is tired. A young child may appear wide awake and excited when in fact she is overstimulated, overtired and ready for bed.
- ◎ If a child has learnt to settle with certain behaviours or a dummy she may find it difficult to do so without them.
- ◎ Many young children develop the habit known as 'grazing'. They nibble their way through the day, eating and drinking a snack here and there. This includes breast and bottle feeding. It is easy for parents to become confused about whether their child's disgruntled and unhappy behaviour is due to tiredness or hunger. As a result,

the child is offered food or drink rather than being put to bed because of tiredness.

There are lots of times when parents accidentally give their children 'mixed messages' about sleep. This means that the parents say one thing but do something quite different. This can be confusing for young children as they learn through the repetition and consistency of the messages being given to them. For example, the parent says it is bedtime and yet does not act to ensure that the child goes to bed. They allow other events to delay bedtime for the child. The result is a blurred and confused message for the child, with a number of different meanings. The child may end up thinking any or all of the following:

◎ It's not really bedtime.
◎ The 'other events' that take over are more important than bedtime.
◎ Mum/Dad has not acted on their comment that it's bedtime therefore I can make the decision about when I can go to bed.
◎ I am in command here.
◎ Mum/Dad did not really mean what they said.
◎ The longer I stay up the better.

It is easy to see that if any of these ideas become established in the child's mind it could have a detrimental effect on the settling and sleep patterns for the child and the whole family. If this continues, bedtime will take longer and longer and ultimately will become difficult for both the parents and child.

A situation that commonly occurs is that, on getting ready for bed, the baby or young child is excited by their well-meaning parents, brothers, sisters or visitors. The child will appear then to be wide awake and many parents will feel that their child is not at all tired. Consequently, there may be a tendency to allow the child to stay up a little later. The parents will then have a struggle on their hands to settle the excited and overstimulated child into bed. Babies and young children are often funny and cute but extra stimulation and excitement are best left for times when the child is not tired and is not about to go to bed.

Sometimes loud protests and crying on going to bed result in parents relenting, reading another story, giving another cuddle or drink, or allowing the child to get up. At this point many parents, in desperation, allow their child to sleep in their bed.

As you can see, there are many reasons why young children may have problems with settling and sleep. There are also a variety of techniques which health professionals advocate and parents adopt to help them alter their young child's sleeping pattern. Which technique you use is a matter of personal choice.

The aim of the settling and sleep techniques

The aim and success of these techniques is that they teach children to:

◎ Fall asleep on their own.
◎ Resettle themselves when they wake prematurely or between sleep cycles.
◎ Sleep for longer periods, both day and night.

The techniques have a strong emphasis on providing comfort and reassurance to the young child. We all need security and support, especially when we attempt to alter our behaviour, and young children are no exception. These techniques have been developed with the different developmental ages and stages of babies and young children in mind and are described in the relevant chapters. As babies and children are all individual there will always be small variations in development. The techniques for settling young babies (up to 6 months old) are based on providing comfort and security. After about 6 months babies become more active, alert and mobile. To stay with a baby of this age patting them for a prolonged period of time may further stimulate them, create a sleep association and extend the settling process.

From 6 months, babies begin to develop what is called 'object and person permanence'. This means that they are starting to learn that a person or object has not ceased to exist because it has disappeared from sight. However, because a baby or young child is never left for more than 10 minutes when using the settling techniques, the emphasis is still on providing comfort and reassurance. All this will make more sense when we talk about the techniques in the following chapters.

There are three key elements to achieving change in your child's sleep pattern:

◎ Realistic expectations and knowledge of sleep needs that change as your child progresses through her developmental stages.
◎ Giving your child consistent messages about settling and sleep.
◎ Persistence in using the techniques with your child.

Understanding sleep

Sleep is necessary for the good health, growth and development of children of all ages. A child who sleeps well becomes more settled, happier and easier to read, and as a parent it is easier to know what your child needs.

Tiredness often masks other behaviours. Sleep is also required by adults to enable them to perform their work, parenting and partnering activities in a happy and tolerant frame of mind.

> It's really great that Luke sleeps. Now I can sit down and relax, even watch a movie. **KIRSTY**

To help your baby to establish a good sleeping pattern and to gradually learn the difference between day and night, it is recommended that when settling you:

◎ Close the curtains during the day still allowing natural light into the room.
◎ Close the curtains at night.
◎ Use dimmed lighting at night when attending to your baby's needs,
◎ Eliminate the play component of 'feed, play, sleep' overnight.
◎ Reduce the amount of general stimulation overnight.

How do we sleep?

It is not our purpose to examine the theory of sleep and sleep cycles in detail, however, it is important for parents to understand a few aspects of sleep. The sleep of both adults and children is made up of many sleep cycles. Each sleep cycle consists of two different states. These are Rapid Eye Movement (REM), often called 'light sleep' and non-REM, often called 'deep sleep'. The non-REM state can further be divided into four different stages. To understand and apply the techniques described, it is only necessary to discuss light and deep states of sleep.

Adults have sleep cycles lasting approximately 90 minutes. Babies and young children have much shorter sleep cycles. The sleep cycles of very young babies last about 20–40 minutes. In older babies and young children the sleep cycle lasts about 60 minutes. Between each sleep cycle both children and adults wake or rouse briefly and then resettle to sleep. This is quite normal.

Generally, we are not aware of waking between sleep cycles. In fact, we do not usually wake fully. An adult might turn over, adjust the pillow and resettle quickly back to sleep.

Many children also resettle themselves back to sleep after this brief waking. At the end of a sleep cycle of 20–40 minutes they wake or rouse and, like adults, can resettle themselves back to sleep. However, some children have not learnt how to do this and require help to get back to sleep. They let you know by crying, calling out or coming into your bed. Does this sound familiar to you?

In our work with parents we explore the difference between sleep *associations* and sleep messages.

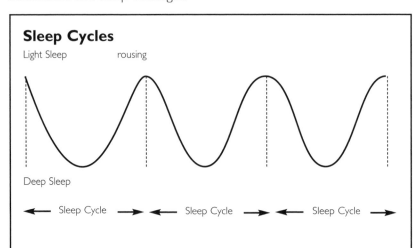

Sleep Cycles

Light Sleep   rousing

Deep Sleep

← Sleep Cycle →   ← Sleep Cycle →   ← Sleep Cycle →

We all sleep in patterns called 'sleep cycles'. During a sleep cycle we begin with the light or Rapid Eye Movement sleep, progressing into deep sleep and back again into light sleep before rousing and either waking or resettling back to sleep. The length of babies' sleep cycles ranges from 20 to 40 minutes. By the time a baby turns 1, the sleep cycles lasts about an hour and an adult sleep cycle is approximately 90 minutes. The most restorative sleep occurs early in the night.

Sleep messages

A sleep message is a process that reinforces the need for self settling by the baby. It involves that establishment of trust between parent and child, it introduces the concept of predictability to the child by using calming repetitive actions, sending messages that it is time for sleep. For example, 'Shh, shh shh'. It is also part of providing comfort and security to your baby.

Sleep associations

If children are unable to resettle themselves to sleep after a sleep cycle is finished, it may be because the circumstances in which they went to sleep are no longer present. On waking, the child may think she needs to be cuddled if she was settled to sleep in this way. She may become distressed and unable to return to sleep.

If a child has a dummy when falling asleep, she may expect it to be there when resettling herself to asleep. If the dummy is lost, the child may wake fully and cry. If she went to sleep lying down with Mum or Dad then wakes to find them absent she may cry through confusion and anxiety. The child may feel that she requires the parent's presence before she can fall back to sleep.

These examples of the links children may develop with sleep are often referred to as sleep associations or sleep connections. The situation that enabled the child to fall asleep needs to be re-created as they wake between sleep cycles. This means that instead of waking briefly and returning to sleep, parental assistance is required. The child will cry, obtain her parents' attention and rely on her parents' assistance to fall asleep again. During the night this results in the child and parents having a disturbed sleep and consequently experiencing all the other feelings associated with sleep deprivation.

During the daytime another scenario develops. The child wakes up after one sleep cycle of 20–40 minutes. Her parents, believing she's had enough sleep, get her out of bed. The child, having had insufficient quality sleep, becomes irritable and unhappy. This may result in unsettled behaviour. Parents may incorrectly believe their child has a feeding or other problem when the real problem is lack of sleep.

Generally, once a child's sleep pattern improves and adequate sleep is attained, an overall improvement will occur in her behaviour.

Sleep for babies and young children

Parents often ask: 'How much sleep does my young child need?' We all have individual needs and the 'feed, play, sleep' pattern provides a useful guide to ensuring that your baby or young child has all her needs met.

A baby will generally require a sleep of at least one hour, or two full sleep cycles, between each feed. If your baby wakes under one hour it is important to try and resettle her. When using the 'feed, play, sleep' pattern, each feed is followed by a play period, which includes cuddling or other activities.

As the baby gets older:

◎ The number of daytime breast or bottle feeds decreases.
◎ The length of time between feeds increases.
◎ A sleep is still required between each feed.
◎ More time is spent interacting and playing before and/or after feeds.
◎ The length of the night sleep increases.
◎ During the night the 'feed, sleep' pattern only is practised.

> Tom [aged 10 months] is now sleeping in his cot all night. This is 100 per cent better than when we were getting up ten times a night. He is a much happier baby. He is crawling around getting into different trouble now! **MANDY**

The chart on page 17 illustrates the 'feed, play, sleep' pattern. As you can see, the amount of time between sleeps lengthens as the baby gets older and she spends more time awake and playing. While your young child still requires a morning and afternoon sleep, the 'feed, play, sleep' pattern is still relevant. When a baby is young, a 'feed' refers to a breast or bottle feed, but as the baby gets older this can also incorporate a drink and food.

Many parents are surprised to learn how much sleep children need and believe their child will never sleep that much. However, after gaining an understanding of sleep and by following the techniques described in this book, they find their children develop improved patterns not only for sleeping but also for behaviour and eating.

Feed, play, sleep chart

Daytime Pattern

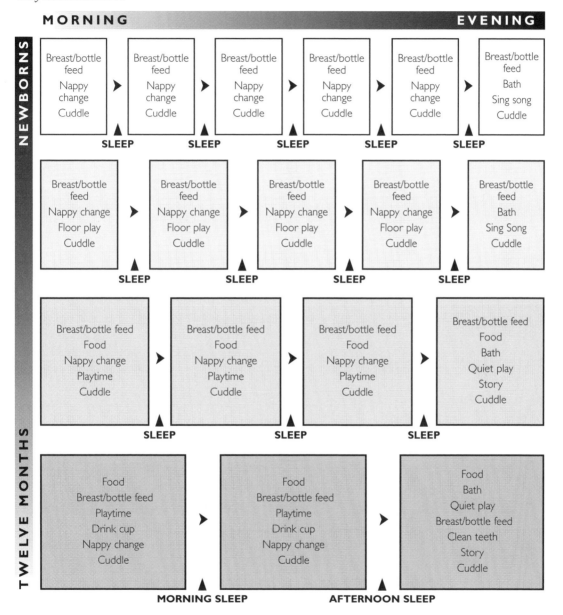

MORNING

EVENING

NEWBORNS

| Breast/bottle feed
Nappy change
Cuddle | ► | Breast/bottle feed
Nappy change
Cuddle | ► | Breast/bottle feed
Nappy change
Cuddle | ► | Breast/bottle feed
Nappy change
Cuddle | ► | Breast/bottle feed
Nappy change
Cuddle | ► | Breast/bottle feed
Bath
Sing song
Cuddle |

▲ SLEEP   ▲ SLEEP   ▲ SLEEP   ▲ SLEEP   ▲ SLEEP

Breast/bottle feed / Nappy change / Floor play / Cuddle ►
Breast/bottle feed / Nappy change / Floor play / Cuddle ►
Breast/bottle feed / Nappy change / Floor play / Cuddle ►
Breast/bottle feed / Nappy change / Floor play / Cuddle ►
Breast/bottle feed / Bath / Sing Song / Cuddle

▲ SLEEP   ▲ SLEEP   ▲ SLEEP   ▲ SLEEP

Breast/bottle feed / Food / Nappy change / Playtime / Cuddle ►
Breast/bottle feed / Food / Nappy change / Playtime / Cuddle ►
Breast/bottle feed / Food / Nappy change / Playtime / Cuddle ►
Breast/bottle feed / Food / Bath / Quiet play / Story / Cuddle

▲ SLEEP   ▲ SLEEP   ▲ SLEEP

TWELVE MONTHS

Food / Breast/bottle feed / Playtime / Drink cup / Nappy change / Cuddle ►
Food / Breast/bottle feed / Playtime / Drink cup / Nappy change / Cuddle ►
Food / Bath / Quiet play / Breast/bottle feed / Clean teeth / Story / Cuddle

▲ MORNING SLEEP   ▲ AFTERNOON SLEEP

Remember: During the night, the feed, sleep pattern only is practised

As baby gets older the number of daytime feeds gradually decreases and she is awake longer. The number of daytime sleeps are reduced and she gradually sleeps longer overnight.

Personal notes

_____

_____

_____

_____

_____

_____

_____

_____

_____

_____

_____

_____

_____

_____

_____

_____

_____

_____

CHAPTER 3

Babies up to 3 months old

General sleep information	21
Infant communication and crying	21
Learn to recognise tired cues	23
Quiet wind down time	24
Getting ready	24
To wrap or not to wrap	25
Settling without wrapping	25
Settling with wrapping	25
Use of dummies	26
Settling your baby	26
Relaxation strategies	27
Baby massage	27
Relaxation bathing	28
Looking after yourself	30
Frequently asked questions	32
Conclusion	32
Personal notes	50
CHARTS	
Weekly feed, play, sleep charts	34
Settling progress chart	42

General sleep information

We know that newborn babies are already very clever and waiting for learning to begin. This happens best through love and nurturing. Your baby receives all of these warm feelings through her sensory pathways, by touch, smell, sound, sight. We know for the last few weeks of your pregnancy, your baby was developing quiet times and active times, practising for after birth. You can probably remember this. This is what we mean by biological rhythms. By responding to your baby's needs, including establishing effective feeding, you will see your baby gradually develop the ability to regulate her own rhythms, including day and night patterns. This usually begins between 2 and 3 months of age and is a special time to get to know your baby, learning to read her cues – and allowing your baby time to get to know you.

During the first few weeks of life it is normal for babies to feed and sleep frequently. For further information about feeding see our book *Eat Right, Don't Fight*.

Some parents ask: 'Can I feed my baby to sleep? If I do this, won't I be creating bad habits and make her dependent on this?' Babies grow so quickly, for many people cuddling and feeding a young baby to sleep is one of the many pleasures of having a new baby. This is fine, do what you feel is right. Many babies will sleep well after they have been cuddled or fed to sleep. However, as time goes by, continued use of these practices can create sleep associations. Sleep associations can create confusion and result in sleeping problems. If babies are always fed to sleep they are not given the opportunity to learn to settle themselves. We recommend that you provide your baby with two or three opportunities to self settle in every 24-hour period. If you are feeling unhappy about your baby's sleeping or behaviour, there are some practical guidelines later in this chapter that may help. Remember, the 'feed, play, sleep' principle discussed in Chapter 2 provides an excellent guide to caring for the needs of babies.

Infant communication and crying

Communication is an example of baby's cleverness, telling us what they need. Through detailed videotaping by researchers, we now know that babies from birth tell us through their body language and vocalisations what they need. For example:

An 'I need a feed' sign may be:

◎ hands to mouth with sucking movements
◎ tight fists over chest or tummy

As her hunger is satisfied she may relax her arms which go down by her side.

An 'I want to play' sign may be:

◎ smiling, vocalising
◎ looking at your face
◎ reaching out to touch you

This is a good time to talk, hold, and play with her.

An 'I need a break' sign may be:

◎ back-arching
◎ fussing
◎ fast-breathing
◎ hand behind ear
◎ looking away

Allow your baby to take a rest or have some time by herself.

An 'I need a sleep' sign may be

◎ changes in facial expression   ◎ jerky movements
◎ minimal movements   ◎ staring
◎ grimacing   ◎ rigid limbs
◎ frowning   ◎ yawning
◎ grizzling   ◎ crying
◎ clenching fists

Time to settle your baby to bed.

Babies can calm themselves on their own, but loud crying is a definite sign from your baby for you to respond. By the time your baby cries, she may no longer be able to wait and will need immediate attention. This is her most potent way of communicating her needs. As above, she may be hungry, want to play, need a break or be tired.

Especially in the early days, however, the reason for crying may not be obvious. Studies have shown that the total time a baby cries each day may rise steadily from birth, peaking at six weeks of age. The crying time may be up to three hours in total during a 24-hour period.

An unsettled period is considered normal and usually occurs in the evening. It is thought this may be due to a newborn's immature nervous system releasing tension build-up from the day. This may range from unsettledness to crying between the space of two feeds. During this time your baby may need more frequent feeding or close body contact. See the section on relaxation, pp. 27–30, for other strategies to try. Later in the evening, and after frequent feeding, your baby may be able to sleep for a longer period of time which can help the day–night patterns emerge. Fortunately, by 2–3 months this unsettled period begins to settle.

As a parent, however, it is hard to listen to your baby cry. If you are concerned in any way, see your doctor or child health nurse.

Jacob [aged 12 weeks] has established a feeding and sleeping pattern and is a much happier child and my husband and I are a lot happier also. LINH

Learn to recognise tired cues

Before discussing techniques and strategies for developing better sleep patterns, it is important that you learn to recognise the 'cues' or 'I need a sleep' signs your baby gives you to indicate tiredness that are listed on p. 22. It may take a little while, as they can easily be mistaken. For example, a baby's jerky leg movements might be interpreted as simple kicking when in fact they may be telling you that they are tired.

When trying to establish improved sleeping patterns, it is important to pick up on the tired cues early. As your baby becomes increasingly tired, her behaviour may become more unsettled and difficult to understand and manage. An overtired baby will be more difficult to settle. So begin to settle your baby to bed when you see a couple of her tired cues.

Quiet wind down time

Before going to bed in her cot, a quiet wind down time will help your baby to relax and learn that it is time for bed. This is the beginning of the settling and sleep process. The quiet wind down time will become part of the relaxing process that your baby learns to associate with sleep and will be a positive, clear signal to your baby that sleep time is imminent. Quiet wind down time may be as simple as enjoying a cuddle, gentle talking or singing a song – it is just a time when you can relax together before she goes into her cot. It needs only to be for a few minutes as it is meant to provide a 'space' between the 'buzz' of the outside world and the restful security of bed. During wind down time, make sure there is minimal stimulation in the room and speak in a quiet, calm voice.

Getting ready

Before you put your baby into her cot, take extra time to make sure she is comfortable. For example:

◎ Prepare the cot
◎ Change her into a clean nappy
◎ Ensure she is not overdressed, which may result in her becoming overheated (see box below)
◎ Remove toys from the cot
◎ Darken the room to decrease stimulation

DRESSING YOUR BABY
A useful rule of thumb is to dress your baby as you would dress yourself. Remember that overheating is a SIDS risk factor and that babies keep cool through their heads. Do not put a baby down to sleep in a hat or bonnet.

To wrap or not to wrap

It is normal for small babies to have some jerky movements when they are in light sleep as well as a startle reflex which is present until they are about 3–4 months old.

Wrapping is a popular method of settling infants as it is thought to provide security as well as minimising the likelihood of sleep disturbance from jerky movements. However, babies generally do settle if they are not wrapped. It just takes a little longer.

Remember, whatever you choose to do, **do not overheat your baby**.

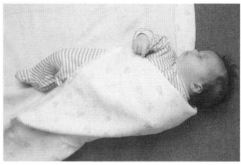

Wrapping: step 1

Settling without wrapping

Tuck your baby in firmly using her bedclothes.

Ensure that she has some movement and is able to put her arms by her sides or above her head.

Settling with wrapping

If you choose to wrap your baby it is important to ensure that your baby is not so tightly wrapped that she cannot move her arms or get her hands to her mouth to comfort herself. Loose wrapping enables some body movement.

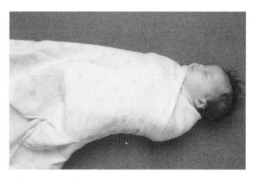

Wrapping: step 2

Wrapping is not recommended after 4 months of age or when your baby starts to roll. For a gradual transition, occasionally place your baby in the cot unwrapped. Alternatively, when your baby approaches this age you could start loosening the wrap or perhaps wrap with one or both arms out. Finally, stop wrapping her and instead tuck her in firmly, as discussed in 'Settling without wrapping', above.

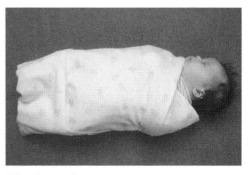

Wrapping: step 3

If the weather is very hot, you may choose to use a very light wrap such as a thin cotton sheet or muslin.

Use of dummies

Using a dummy is an individual choice. It is, however, recommended to wait until breastfeeding is established. Babies need an opportunity to explore their world through their mouths by sucking. Also, sucking helps a baby to establish individual patterns including self settling. This is achieved through feeding and sucking of hands and fingers. If you do choose to use a dummy, it is recommended that you provide your baby with 2–3 opportunities in every 24-hour period to settle without it.

Newborn babies have a normal reflex known as 'extension reflex' or 'tongue thrust reflex'. This thrusting action may cause your baby to push her dummy out. If she continues to push the dummy out, don't persist with replacing it. A dummy must not be dipped in any substance and given to a baby to settle.

Settling your baby

When your baby is ready for sleep, place her in her cot, awake. Place her on her back according to SIDS recommendations (see box below), say 'Goodnight' and leave the room.

Give your baby the chance to go to sleep by herself – babies can calm themselves. If she cries, wait 20–30 seconds then go back into the room as she may need some help to calm down. Start some gentle stroking or patting while she is on her back to quieten and relax her. One soothing action at a time for up to 5 minutes will work best.

As you continue to pat or stroke your baby, she may reach a crying peak (see p. 54) and then quieten. We recommend you stay as long as she is crying. Remember, your baby may have an unsettled period each day.

SUDDEN INFANT DEATH SYNDROME (SIDS) RECOMMENDATIONS

From birth:

1. Put baby on back to sleep

2. Do not overheat your baby, especially the hands and face

3. Cigarette smoke is bad for babies

Relaxation strategies

Baby massage

Baby masssage can be a useful way to:

◎ Relax an unsettled baby
◎ Give your baby the opportunity to enjoy being touched. Sometimes young babies become upset when they are undressed and massage may help reduce this
◎ Allow a parent or caregiver to spend time interacting with and enjoying the baby

Getting ready

Choose a time that is convenient, such as 30 minutes after a feed. Allow about 15–20 minutes. You may wish to take the phone off the hook so you won't be disturbed. Collect the articles you will need:

◎ Towel
◎ Clothes
◎ Nappy
◎ Oil (Use an edible oil such as almond oil, not baby oil or the commercially available scented massage oils. Edible oils do not contain the perfume and chemicals that some other types of oil do. Some oil will be absorbed through the baby's skin and she may lick some of it off.)

Starting the massage

◎ Ensure there are no direct cold draughts near your baby.
◎ Sit in a comfortable position. Completely undress your baby and lie her on a towel. Position her on her back so that you are able to look at her and talk to her. Reassure her and tell her what you are doing.
◎ Pour some oil on your hands and rub your hands together to warm. Stroke your baby using firm but gentle pressure. Using too light a touch may tickle her!
◎ Don't worry about what part of the body to massage first. Try different ways until you find what the baby likes. Don't forget to include her arms, hands, legs, feet and face.

- The massage should be relaxing and enjoyable. If the baby becomes cold or upset, finish the massage.
- Most of the oil will be absorbed through the baby's skin during the massage. This will act as a moisturiser. It is not necessary for the baby to be bathed afterwards, but she may also find a relaxation bath enjoyable.
- There is no age limit on baby massage. A baby as young as a few days old can be massaged. Older children also enjoy the contact and close interaction achieved through massage, although they might be more ticklish.

Relaxation bathing

A gentle bath helps soothe and relax an unsettled baby. It is most suitable for babies aged from newborn to 4 months. Bathing your baby helps develop your confidence and is enjoyable for both baby and parents or caregiver. To give a relaxation bath, first collect the articles you will need for bathing:

- Towels
- Change mat
- Clothes
- Nappy
- Face washer, bath oil, soap, etc. (You will only need these if you are also washing your baby.)

To aid relaxation, the water needs to be deep enough to allow the baby to explore the space around her and feel the effects of floating. To achieve this, fill an adult bath to three-quarters full or fill a baby bath as close to full as possible. (Remember, don't try to carry a full baby bath as you could easily hurt your back.)

The temperature of the water needs to be as warm as a bath you would have yourself (approximately 38° Celsius). The water should feel warm when tested with the inside of your wrist. Ensure that both taps have been turned off before placing the baby in the water. Lower the baby into the bath in the conventional manner, supporting the back of her head with the inside of your wrist. Don't be surprised if she cries when she is undressed and placed in the bath. (If this happens, next time try bathing her while she is wearing her singlet.)

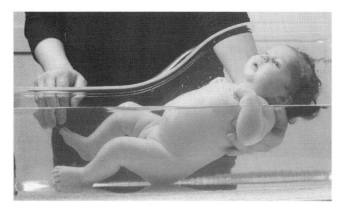

Relaxation bath with baby on back

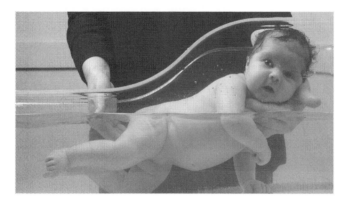

Relaxation bath with baby on front

The relaxation bath seems to work best with the baby on her tummy. If you don't feel confident turning your baby over in the bath this is okay, as many babies will still be able to relax on their back. The most important thing is for you to feel confident. The baby needs to feel supported and safe in the water and able to stretch, explore and relax. If you are going to turn your baby over, do remember that wet babies are slippery so take your time and do this carefully.

Remember to keep your baby's face clear of the water. The baby may be calm and relaxed or may explore the space and volume of the bath by making long sweeping movements with her hands or by kicking her legs. She may even fall asleep.

While bathing her, reassure and talk to her so that she feels secure. She may remain immersed in the bath as long as you are both enjoying it, but finish the bath if she becomes cold or upset.

When lifting the baby out of the bath, support her head and neck and lift her from under her tummy or you could turn her onto her back and lift her out normally.

Relaxation bathing may be repeated as often as is needed or wanted. Parents may also enjoy having a bath with their baby or older children.

Looking after yourself

Do you remember the highs and lows of energy and activity that you experienced while you were pregnant? Do you remember being overcome by tiredness early in your pregnancy but having increased energy later on, perhaps finding yourself cleaning madly? It seemed that your body had a mind of its own, telling you what you needed. Now too, your body knows what it needs, so listen to it. These needs may include:

- ◎ Rest
- ◎ Reassurance
- ◎ Recuperation
- ◎ Relaxation
- ◎ Recharge

You may also remember times in your pregnancy of mixed thoughts and emotions. These may return after having your baby. By now you may have experienced the baby blues. You may need to make decisions about your baby; you may feel a great sense of responsibility and protectiveness – even preoccupation. Now more than ever, let your head and your heart find a balance with each other. Listen to both!

Childbirth is often talked of as a rite of passage. For many cultures, this entails the mother and baby staying indoors for a required length of time, helping to establish feeding and encourage recuperation, supported by the family. We could learn from these cultures in many ways. Sometimes we may expect too much from ourselves during this highly sensitive recuperation phase and time of change. At the very least, try to accept offers of help as gestures of support.

Finally, ask yourself: 'if I were my best friend, what would I say to look after myself'?' and write down a list of ideas. For example, one idea might be: 'I will aim for a 3-hour block of sleep when I first go to bed at night.' As research shows you can then cope better with waking through the rest of the night.

Ideas for looking after myself

Frequently asked questions

Should I drop the cot sides every time I go in to settle?

We recommend that you always leave the cot sides up to give a clear sleep message. Place your hands through the cot sides to settle.

Will my baby get a flat head if she sleeps on her back all the time?

Sleeping on her back is the safest position for your baby. Some babies do get a flat spot on the back of their head, however, the shape of the head continues to change as they grow and develop. Head shapes are influenced by genetics.

Tummy time during floor play provides opportunities for your baby to try different head positions, which gradually your baby will start to enjoy.

If you are concerned about the shape of the baby's head, discuss this with your health professional.

Should I offer my baby a dummy?

Using a dummy is an individual choice. There is no need to introduce a dummy if it is not already being used.

Sometimes it seems that a sleep problem is due to a dummy falling out of the baby's mouth. Sucking on the dummy has become a sleep association and the problem is that she cannot replace it herself. This means that she will rely on you to put it back so that she can resettle.

See Chapter 4 for more FAQs.

Conclusion

An 'older and wiser' new parent will tell you that flexibility is the key to these early days of caring for a new baby. The techniques that may calm a baby at one time of day may not work at another. This may seem confusing, but the times it is working are the times your baby is learning. The other times she is learning that you are there for her.

Remember that by 2–3 months of age, babies begin to respond to differences between day and night as their biological rhythms develop. The evening unsettled period may decrease and your baby may begin to sleep for a longer period at night. We know that introducing a 'feed, play, sleep' pattern will help build on this natural process. This pattern will also help babies of this age who haven't yet developed these rhythms.

Weekly feed, play, sleep chart

It is easy to feel that you are up all night with your baby, or that she is constantly feeding or crying. It may be helpful to have an accurate picture of your baby's feed, play and sleep pattern, so that you can maintain some perspective during stressful times. Completing this chart will also help you see the progress you are making with your baby. To fill in the chart, shade the area to show when your baby is asleep on each day. When your baby is awake, leave the spaces clear. When she has been fed, write an F in the box. Try to continue filling out the chart for 2–3 weeks. You will begin to see patterns in your baby's life.

	6 AM	7 AM	8 AM	9 AM	10 AM	11 AM	12 MD	1 PM	2 PM	3 PM	4 PM	
MONDAY												
TUESDAY												
WEDNESDAY												
THURSDAY												
FRIDAY												
SATURDAY												
SUNDAY												

■ DENOTES SLEEPING
☐ DENOTES AWAKE
F DENOTES FEED

	5 PM	6 PM	7 PM	8 PM	9 PM	10 PM	11 PM	12 MN	1 AM	2 AM	3 AM	4 AM	5 AM

Weekly feed, play, sleep chart

	6 AM	7 AM	8 AM	9 AM	10 AM	11 AM	12 MD	1 PM	2 PM	3 PM	4 PM	
MONDAY												
TUESDAY												
WEDNESDAY												
THURSDAY												
FRIDAY												
SATURDAY												
SUNDAY												

■ DENOTES SLEEPING
□ DENOTES AWAKE
F DENOTES FEED

	5 PM	6 PM	7 PM	8 PM	9 PM	10 PM	11 PM	12 MN	1 AM	2 AM	3 AM	4 AM	5 AM

Weekly feed, play, sleep chart

	6 AM	7 AM	8 AM	9 AM	10 AM	11 AM	12 MD	1 PM	2 PM	3 PM	4 PM	
MONDAY												
TUESDAY												
WEDNESDAY												
THURSDAY												
FRIDAY												
SATURDAY												
SUNDAY												

■ DENOTES SLEEPING
□ DENOTES AWAKE
F DENOTES FEED

	5 PM	6 PM	7 PM	8 PM	9 PM	10 PM	11 PM	12 MN	1 AM	2 AM	3 AM	4 AM	5 AM

Weekly feed, play, sleep chart

	6 AM	7 AM	8 AM	9 AM	10 AM	11 AM	12 MD	1 PM	2 PM	3 PM	4 PM	
MONDAY												
TUESDAY												
WEDNESDAY												
THURSDAY												
FRIDAY												
SATURDAY												
SUNDAY												

■ DENOTES SLEEPING
□ DENOTES AWAKE
F DENOTES FEED

	5 PM	6 PM	7 PM	8 PM	9 PM	10 PM	11 PM	12 MN	1 AM	2 AM	3 AM	4 AM	5 AM

Settling progress chart

When you fill in this chart over a 24-hour period, it will allow you to see how much time you are spending settling and resettling your baby. Over a few days you will ideally see that the time spent settling is reducing. Sometimes it is easy to forget how long you were spending and how the situation has improved. When you look at your progress you will realise how far you have come!

TIME OVER 24 HOURS

	6 AM	7 AM	8 AM	9 AM	10 AM	11 AM	12 MD	1 PM	2 PM	3 PM	4 PM	
0												
5												
10												
15												
20												
25												
30												
35												
40												
45												
50												
55												
60												
TOTAL												

MINUTES SPENT SETTLING

	5 PM	6 PM	7 PM	8 PM	9 PM	10 PM	11 PM	12 MN	1 AM	2 AM	3 AM	4 AM	5 AM

Settling progress chart

TIME OVER 24 HOURS

	6 AM	7 AM	8 AM	9 AM	10 AM	11 AM	12 MD	1 PM	2 PM	3 PM	4 PM	
0												
5												
10												
15												
20												
25												
30												
35												
40												
45												
50												
55												
60												
TOTAL												

MINUTES SPENT SETTLING

	5 PM	6 PM	7 PM	8 PM	9 PM	10 PM	11 PM	12 MN	1 AM	2 AM	3 AM	4 AM	5 AM

Settling progress chart

TIME OVER 24 HOURS

	6 AM	7 AM	8 AM	9 AM	10 AM	11 AM	12 MD	1 PM	2 PM	3 PM	4 PM	
0												
5												
10												
15												
20												
25												
30												
35												
40												
45												
50												
55												
60												
TOTAL												

MINUTES SPENT SETTLING

	5 PM	6 PM	7 PM	8 PM	9 PM	10 PM	11 PM	12 MN	1 AM	2 AM	3 AM	4 AM	5 AM

Settling progress chart

TIME OVER 24 HOURS

	6 AM	7 AM	8 AM	9 AM	10 AM	11 AM	12 MD	1 PM	2 PM	3 PM	4 PM	
0												
5												
10												
15												
20												
25												
30												
35												
40												
45												
50												
55												
60												
TOTAL												

MINUTES SPENT SETTLING

	5 PM	6 PM	7 PM	8 PM	9 PM	10 PM	11 PM	12 MN	1 AM	2 AM	3 AM	4 AM	5 AM

Personal notes

_____

_____

_____

_____

_____

_____

_____

_____

_____

_____

_____

_____

_____

_____

_____

_____

_____

CHAPTER 4

Babies 3–6 months old

General sleep information	53
About crying	53
Signs of tiredness	54
Quiet wind down time	55
To wrap or not to wrap	55
Settling your baby	56
Getting started	56
Pre-sleep signs	58
Looking after yourself	60
Points to remember	61
Frequently asked questions	62
Conclusion	65
Management plan	66
Personal notes	86

CHARTS
Settling flow chart	59
Weekly feed, play, sleep chart	70
Settling progress chart	78

General sleep information

Some babies will sleep well after they have been cuddled or fed to sleep. However, if babies are always fed or cuddled to sleep and are not given the opportunity to learn to settle themselves, they may develop sleep associations and difficulties in self settling. We recommend that you provide your baby with 2–3 opportunities to self settle in a 24-hour period.

You may have found that your baby is not completing feeds, is feeding continuously and/or is wakeful or irritable if she is not having enough sleep. If you are feeling unhappy about your baby's sleeping or behaviour, here are some practical guidelines that may help. Remember, the 'feed, play, sleep' principle provides an excellent guide to caring for the needs of babies.

About crying

As you begin to alter sleep patterns, your baby may respond to the changes with crying. Crying is a way of communicating with you. As a baby gradually learns what you are teaching them, the crying will lessen and may cease. Babies cry for many reasons including hunger, tiredness or discomfort. Sometimes the reason is not obvious to us. Many parents find it hard to listen to their baby cry.

By 3 months of age, crying communicates a more specific need to parents and caregivers. If a baby cries during the settling process her cry usually builds up to a peak (see the diagram, p. 54). Once the crying has peaked she will often have much shorter, less intense bursts of crying. The baby then begins to quieten before settling. The time taken from the beginning of crying to when a baby settles and is relaxed can vary. Many parents find listening to their baby's cry too distressing to allow them to reach this peak, but even though the intense crying period may make you feel uncomfortable it is important to continue the settling strategies.

By being consistent with the settling strategies you give your baby clear and consistent messages that you want her to go to sleep. This will help her through the learning process. Try not to focus on the crying because it will stop. Focus on giving her clear, positive sleep messages and listen for the change in the crying pattern. If you become too distressed by her crying and feel like stopping the settling process, think of ways

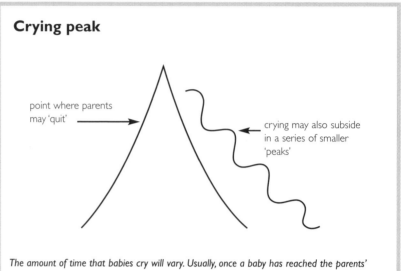

Crying peak

point where parents may 'quit' →

← crying may also subside in a series of smaller 'peaks'

The amount of time that babies cry will vary. Usually, once a baby has reached the parents' 'quitting point' her cry will peak within five minutes. She will then have shorter, less intense bouts of crying until she settles. The 'crying peak' concept only applies to babies up to the age of 12 months. After this time children are able to sustain their crying for longer and may not have a defined 'crying peak'.

that you can remain calm to continue (see 'Looking after yourself' p. 60).

Babies who have developed sleep associations can learn to settle themselves to sleep. By being with your baby through the crying peak and giving her comforting sleep messages, she will learn to settle herself.

If you are implementing this change by yourself or with your partner, think about some things that will help you cope through this time. We will give you some suggestions later on (see pp. 60–61). Often, just being aware and understanding of your baby's crying patterns will help you to continue.

Signs of tiredness

Before discussing techniques and strategies for developing better sleep patterns, it is important that you learn to recognise the 'cues' or 'I need a sleep' signs your baby gives you to indicate tiredness. These may include:

◎ Changes in facial expression
◎ Grimacing
◎ Jerky movements
◎ Staring

- Minimal movements and little activity
- Frowning
- Resisting distraction
- Yawning
- Crying
- Seeking to be picked up
- Rigid limbs
- Grizzling
- Sucking
- Clenching fists

It may take a little while to recognise these as tired cues as they can easily be mistaken. For example, a baby's jerky leg movements might be interpreted as simple kicking when in fact they may be tired!

When trying to establish improved sleeping patterns, it is important to pick up on the tired cues early. As your baby becomes increasingly tired, her behaviour may become more unsettled and difficult to understand and manage. An overtired baby will be more difficult to settle. So begin to settle your baby to bed when you see a couple of her tired cues.

Quiet wind down time

Before going to bed in her cot, a quiet wind down time will help your baby to relax and learn that it is time for bed. This is the beginning of the settling and sleep process. The quiet wind down time will become part of the relaxing process that your baby learns to associate with sleep and be a positive clear signal to your baby that sleep time is imminent. It may be as simple as enjoying a cuddle, gentle talking or singing a song – it is just a time when you can relax together before she goes into her cot. The aim is to decrease stimulation by using one calming repetitive action, such as repeating the same song or story.

The length of the wind down time will depend on the activity level of your baby. For a very active baby, start the wind down time as soon as you see a couple of tired signs. The wind down time is meant to provide a 'space' between the 'buzz' of the outside world and the restful security of bed, so make sure there is minimal stimulation in the room and speak in a quiet, calm voice.

To wrap or not to wrap

It is not recommended to wrap your baby once she reaches 4 months of age or has started to roll.

Settling your baby

When your baby is ready for sleep, place her in her cot, awake. Place her on her back according to SIDS recommendations (see p. 26). If she is over 4 months, tuck her in firmly, ensuring she has some movement and is able to put her arms by her sides or above her head. Say 'Goodnight' and leave the room.

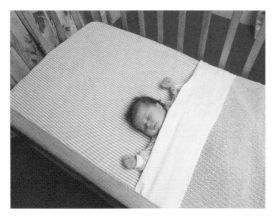

Positioning baby in a cot with hands out

Give your baby the chance to go to sleep by herself. If she cries, wait 20–30 seconds then go back into the room. Now is the time to start the settling techniques. The techniques you choose will depend on you, your time and the baby's response.

Use the settling techniques to comfort, quieten and relax your baby. However, leave her awake so she can learn to settle to sleep herself. Your aim is to create conditions and establish sleep associations that will still be there when your baby wakes between sleep cycles. She will then be able to resettle herself.

Getting started

Make sure you are comfortable. Put on your dressing gown if it is the middle of the night and have a stool or cushion to sit on when you are settling or resettling your baby. We recommend that you always leave the cot side up and put your hands through the bars to settle. See also the suggestions in 'Looking after yourself', pp. 60–61.

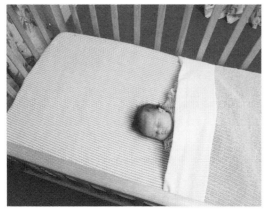

Positioning baby in a cot with hands tucked in

Begin with some gentle long strokes of her body while she is on her back. If after 5 minutes she has not responded, you could now turn her onto her side, facing away from you.

Another technique that can be used when your baby has been turned onto her side is to gently, but firmly, place your hand on her shoulder. With your other hand cupped, pat her gently and slowly on the bottom or thigh. To cup your hand properly, hold your fingers close together and make a cup of your hand as you would do to scoop up water. This ensures that the patting motion is controlled and you will not pat too firmly. Keep the patting to a slow rhythm to help her wind down. You may find it helpful to count as you pat or sing a song quietly to her or in your head.

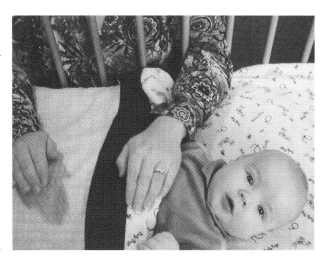

Patting with a cupped hand

Double patting may also be helpful. To do this, continue patting your baby's bottom or thigh and also pat her shoulder with your other hand. Alternate the pats in a rhythmic way. You may want to sing a slow nursery rhyme or song (either aloud or in your head) to help you get started. Slow your hand movements down as your baby starts to settle and relax – watch for the pre-sleep signs (see box, p 58). Once she is quiet, you may like to leave your hands on her without patting for a few seconds before you remove them. Gently turn her onto her back before you leave the room when she is calm and quiet but not asleep or wait until she is asleep then turn her onto her back. This is part of the process of teaching her to go to sleep by herself. Settling your baby on her side is a short term strategy. Ultimately she will be able to go to sleep by herself when you place her into her cot awake, on her back.

Other techniques that you could use to settle and comfort your baby include:
◎ Gentle stroking of her forehead
◎ Soft music or singing
◎ Placing your hands reassuringly on her shoulder and bottom
◎ Sshing

Keep your talking to a minimum. Gentle 'sshing' or saying 'go to sleep, go to sleep' will give clear sleep messages and help you both to relax.

Use the settling techniques to comfort, quieten and relax your baby. However leave her awake so she can learn to settle to sleep herself. Your

PRE-SLEEP SIGNS

When you are using the settling techniques, watch for your baby's pre-sleep signs. These signs indicate it is time to leave her and let her settle herself to sleep. Look and listen for signs such as:

- Body becoming relaxed
- Change in crying
- Fluttering of her eyelids
- Sobbing and sighing
- Tuneful hums and groans

aim is to create conditions that will still be there when your baby wakes between sleep cycles. She will then be able to resettle herself.

If your baby is crying intensely and you have been using one type of settling technique for more than five minutes, try changing to a different technique. If your baby continues to cry and doesn't respond after you have tried two or three more settling strategies (approximately 15–20 minutes), you could both have a break. Give her a cuddle and a feed if needed, or a quiet play on the floor, then try to settle her again when she shows you her 'tired cues'.

If your baby settles but wakes under an hour resettle her using the above techniques. When she wakes and cries, quietly go to her. Use a soothing voice, retuck and use settling techniques until she calms again. See the flow chart of the settling techniques used for babies up to 6 months old, opposite.

Settling flow chart
For babies up to 6 months old

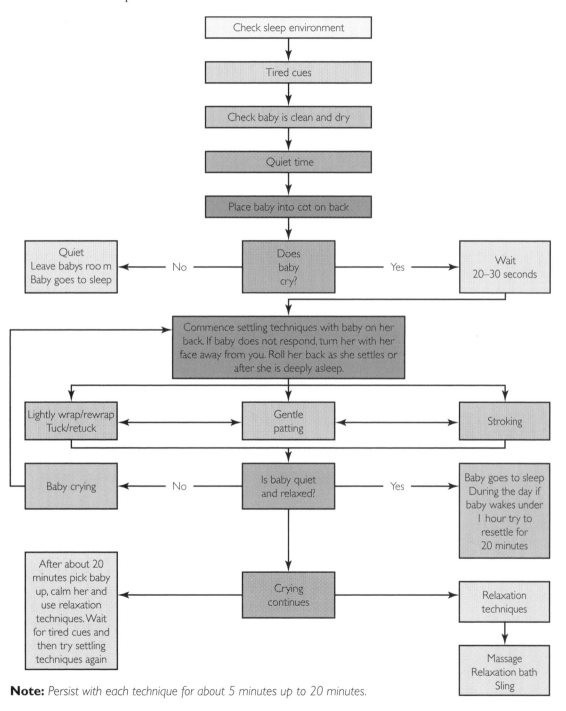

Note: *Persist with each technique for about 5 minutes up to 20 minutes.*

Looking after yourself

Helping your baby to establish an improved sleeping pattern may not be easy. Sometimes it is hard to change. Even though you really want to alter your baby's sleeping patterns, new ideas and strategies can feel unfamiliar and sometimes it can seem easier to revert to what you already know. But just thinking about change means that you are already halfway there. These methods are very successful and redirecting your energy to change sleeping patterns will be well worth it for you, your baby and your family.

While you are using settling techniques, it may be helpful to use some distraction or diversion yourself. These can include:

◎ Using headphones
◎ Practising deep breathing exercises or relaxation techniques
◎ Learning a new song to sing

You may already know some relaxation strategies that you have used successfully at other times in your life. It may also be helpful to:

◎ Plan for support during the process
◎ Talk to someone about how you are feeling
◎ Reward yourself for any progress that you make

Like adults, babies are individuals and vary in their response to change. Experience has shown that a struggle to achieve a new pattern is rarely fruitless, so hang in there! On particular days and nights it may be really hard to keep going and you may need to take time out. You could modify the process but try to keep within the basic principles. It is most important that changing her sleeping patterns is manageable for you, but recognise that modifying the process may result in slower progress. This may be preferable to giving up.

It is important for all the family that you do not keep going if the process is too stressful or if it is not okay for you. It may be necessary for your partner or a friend to take over. You may decide that the time is not right for change in your lives now or that you need more support to implement the strategies. None of these is a bad reflection on you but rather a positive acknowledgement of the importance of looking after yourself and being able to recognise your limits. This is far healthier than getting angry or punishing yourself or your baby.

It is also important to congratulate both yourself and your baby. Tell her that you are both making great progress and how proud you are of her. Don't forget to tell yourself as well!

Be aware that you may have unexpected feelings regarding separation from your baby. You may have been used to holding and cuddling your baby for long periods of time in your efforts to get her to sleep. Think about something that you would like to do with the new time you will have when your baby is sleeping.

Points to remember

◎ As all babies and parents are different, adjust this method to suit your family. Take into consideration your baby's temperament, health and her developmental age.

◎ Talk to someone about the support that you feel you will need to follow the process through.

◎ Start the sleep behaviour changes when you know you can put other activities aside to focus on you and your baby, and when you know you can see the program through.

◎ Help your baby establish an improved sleeping pattern when she is well.

◎ Because babies learn by repetition, consistency and persistence will bring change.

◎ Watch for signs of tiredness.

◎ Have a quiet wind down time with your baby before settling.

◎ Place your baby into her cot awake.

◎ Use settling strategies to quieten your baby only, not to put her to sleep.

◎ Aim for a sleep of at least 1 hour between each feed. (This is for your baby but you can sleep too if you want!)

◎ Resettle your baby if she sleeps for less than 1 hour.

◎ Be aware that you may have unexpected feelings regarding separation from your baby if you are used to her being awake for long periods of time. Think about what you might like to do with the extra time you will have while she is sleeping.

◎ The long-term aim is for your baby to be able to settle and resettle herself to sleep. You can teach her to do this.

- ◎ If there are times when your baby does not settle or resettle, don't feel bad or think it has been a waste of time. The repetition of the settling techniques is valuable and your baby will eventually learn.
- ◎ Reward and congratulate yourself.
- ◎ You can do it!

Frequently asked questions

My baby becomes more irritated by hands-on techniques. What will I do?

If your baby becomes increasingly upset when you are using hands-on techniques you could try placing one hand on her buttocks and one on her shoulder without movement. This will help her feel secure. Continue to say: 'Ssh, ssh'. When she relaxes, lighten the hand on her buttocks until you can remove it. Then do the same with the other hand.

I have tried everything and my baby just won't settle. What do you suggest?

If you feel that you have tried the settling strategies and your baby is overtired and will not settle, get her up and try one of the following:

- ◎ Give your baby a massage and/or a relaxation bath (see pp. 27–30).
- ◎ During the day, put your baby in the pram and take her for a walk.
- ◎ Use a baby sling.

Remember that your baby will not always respond to the settling strategies. You are both learning something new and it will take practice and repetition to make it work. Each settling is not about winning and losing, it is about making small steps of progress towards your goal of improving your baby's sleeping patterns.

If my baby is sick what will happen to her sleeping pattern?

During illness, normal sleeping patterns can be disrupted. The baby may wake more frequently due to discomfort, pain or because she needs extra feeds. Young children, like adults, can't be expected to sleep well if they are ill. When she is well again, however, the sleep disruptions may remain. If they do, restart the settling techniques to help your baby re-establish her normal healthy sleeping patterns.

My baby is nearly 6 months old. She takes longer and longer to settle and at times does not respond to the settling strategies. What will I do?
Think about your baby's activity level and length of quiet wind down time. Try starting this a little earlier when you see the first tired signs. Falling asleep can be harder for your baby if she is overtired.

What do my other children do when I am settling my baby?
Explain to your other children what you are doing in terms they can understand. Try to occupy them, for example:

◎ Keep some special toys for them to play with during this time.
◎ Suggest they 'settle' a favourite doll.
◎ Ask another person to be with them.
◎ Tape their favourite television show and encourage them to watch it while settling your baby.
◎ Alternatively, they might like to listen to a music or story tape.

Once you have settled your baby, thank your other children for letting you settle her undisturbed and spend a few minutes with them. They will be more likely to help you in this way again.

Different strategies will work at different times and you will need to be creative and flexible.

I am returning to work and my baby is going to childcare. What will I do?
Discuss the changes that you are planning to make to your baby's settling and sleeping pattern with the childcare centre. Some centres will try to continue with the same strategies but many will find it difficult because of the number of babies that they are looking after. Continue using the techniques whenever you are with your baby. It may take a little longer for them to be effective but with consistency and patience you and your baby will benefit.

> Daniel [aged 6 months] is just amazing. He sleeps well during the day and is beginning to sleep all night. Even when he had croup and a bad cold it had very little effect on everything. I just spent the night in his room with him. **MARIA**

I am unsure how to lead a normal life while I am changing my baby's patterns. Do I need to stay at home until this has happened?

Aim to begin using the techniques when you have a few days at home and can follow through with your plan. If you do have to go out, try to arrange appointments when you think that your baby will be awake. If you need to be out for longer, organise appointments for only half a day instead of the whole day. Your baby will be able to sleep at home for some of the day. Your baby may be overtired when you get home and you may have to persevere with the techniques a little bit longer. If you are able to settle your baby when you are out, aim to follow through with the techniques you've been using at home. This will not always be possible so don't be too hard on yourself.

I think that my baby's dummy has become a sleep association but am unsure how to get rid of it.

There are three ways that you can work on this issue.

Firstly, if your baby has a dummy in her mouth all the time you can limit its use to bedtime only. Remember that babies learn to talk by making noises and gurgling. They may also settle themselves to sleep while making these noises. A dummy can restrict this process.

The second way is to get rid of the dummy completely.

Thirdly, take a more gradual approach: don't offer your baby her dummy when she first goes to bed; instead, wait 1–2 minutes into the settling until you give it to her. You may find she will start settling without it.

Should I drop the cot sides every time I go in to settle?

We recommend that you always leave the cot sides up to give a clear sleep message. Place your hands through the cot sides to settle.

Will my baby get a flat head if she sleeps on her back all of the time?

Sleeping on the back is the safest position for your baby according to SIDS recommendations (p. 26). Some babies do get a flat spot on the back of the head, however, the shape continues to change as they grow and develop. Head shapes are influenced by genetics. Floor play, including tummy time, provides opportunities for your baby to enjoy different head positions. If you are concerned about the shape of your baby's head, see your health professional.

Conclusion

Parents who consistently use age-appropriate settling strategies will usually see an improvement in their baby's sleep pattern by the end of the first week. However, always keep in mind that it may take a little longer to see an even greater improvement. It can take time to change behaviour that has been occurring for a long time.

Often parents also see an improvement in other aspects of their baby's behaviour once a good sleep pattern is established. This can include more effective feeding, being happier when awake and an improvement generally in their interactions with those around them.

You may find that your baby reverts to a disrupted sleeping pattern after a change or illness occurs. Sometimes a change in sleeping behaviour can be a short term development. Generally your baby will respond very quickly to the settling techniques if you need to use them again. Remember, it is important to be persistent and consistent. It is hard work but it will prove to be a positive investment of time and energy and will help everyone to get a rest during the day and a more settled night.

Management plan

The following questions may be useful to consider before you commence the settling techniques with your baby during the day or night. It can be difficult trying to negotiate with your partner/support person when you are both tired and stressed. If you are planning to implement changes it is important that you both agree with what you are going to do. You are more likely to succeed if you are consistent with the techniques and strategies discussed. If you decide to implement these changes by yourself you will still find the following questions helpful.

Think about the questions and write down some responses. There may be other questions that you would like to add that are important to you.

Sleeping environment

Where is your baby going to sleep during this process?

_____

_____

_____

Where are your other children going to sleep?

_____

_____

_____

If your baby uses a dummy

Are you going to stop the use of the dummy immediately?

_____

_____

Are you going to limit the use of the dummy?

_____

_____

Settling

Who is going to be responsible for settling?

_____

_____

a) During the day?

_____

_____

_____

b) During the night?

_____

_____

_____

At what time will this responsibility change?

_____

_____

What will your other children do while you are settling your baby?

_____

_____

_____

Looking after yourself

What strategies are you going to use to support you through the settling? (For example: earphones, music.)

_____

_____

_____

Who is involved with your child that you may need to talk to about the changes that you plan to make? (For example: childcare worker, friends, family, neighbours.)

_____

_____

_____

If you are feeling cross or frustrated, what will you do or who can you talk to?

_____

_____

_____

Who will be there to give you a break if you need one?

_____

_____

_____

What can you do for yourself as a reward for the changes that you have made?

_____

_____

_____

Weekly feed, play, sleep chart

It is easy to feel that you are up all night with your baby, or that she is constantly feeding or crying. It may be helpful to have an accurate picture of your baby's feed, play and sleep pattern, so that you can maintain some perspective during stressful times. Completing this chart will also help you see the progress you are making with your baby. To fill in the chart, shade the area to show when your baby is asleep on each day. When your baby is awake, leave the spaces clear. When she has been fed, write an F in the box. Try to continue filling out the chart for 2–3 weeks. You will begin to see patterns in your baby's life.

		6 AM	7 AM	8 AM	9 AM	10 AM	11 AM	12 MD	1 PM	2 PM	3 PM	4 PM	
25/1	MONDAY	F	▓	F	▓		F	▓		F small	▓	
26/1	TUESDAY	▓	F		▓	▓	F	▓	F	▓	▓	▓	
27/1	WEDNESDAY	▓	F	▓	▓	▓	F						
28/1	THURSDAY												
29/1	FRIDAY												
30/1	SATURDAY												
31/1	SUNDAY												

■ DENOTES SLEEPING
□ DENOTES AWAKE
F DENOTES FEED

5 PM	6 PM	7 PM	8 PM	9 PM	10 PM	11 PM	12 MN	1 AM	2 AM	3 AM	4 AM	5 AM
F small		F	calming	F				F				
F	F	← calming hard →	F			F				F		

Weekly feed, play, sleep chart

	6 AM	7 AM	8 AM	9 AM	10 AM	11 AM	12 MD	1 PM	2 PM	3 PM	4 PM	
MONDAY												
TUESDAY												
WEDNESDAY												
THURSDAY												
FRIDAY												
SATURDAY												
SUNDAY												

■ DENOTES SLEEPING
☐ DENOTES AWAKE
F DENOTES FEED

	5 PM	6 PM	7 PM	8 PM	9 PM	10 PM	11 PM	12 MN	1 AM	2 AM	3 AM	4 AM	5 AM

Weekly feed, play, sleep chart

	6 AM	7 AM	8 AM	9 AM	10 AM	11 AM	12 MD	1 PM	2 PM	3 PM	4 PM	
MONDAY												
TUESDAY												
WEDNESDAY												
THURSDAY												
FRIDAY												
SATURDAY												
SUNDAY												

■ DENOTES SLEEPING
☐ DENOTES AWAKE
F DENOTES FEED

	5 PM	6 PM	7 PM	8 PM	9 PM	10 PM	11 PM	12 MN	1 AM	2 AM	3 AM	4 AM	5 AM

Weekly feed, play, sleep chart

	6 AM	7 AM	8 AM	9 AM	10 AM	11 AM	12 MD	1 PM	2 PM	3 PM	4 PM	
MONDAY												
TUESDAY												
WEDNESDAY												
THURSDAY												
FRIDAY												
SATURDAY												
SUNDAY												

■ DENOTES SLEEPING
☐ DENOTES AWAKE
F DENOTES FEED

	5 PM	6 PM	7 PM	8 PM	9 PM	10 PM	11 PM	12 MN	1 AM	2 AM	3 AM	4 AM	5 AM

Settling progress chart

When you fill in this chart over a 24-hour period, it will allow you to see how much time you are spending settling and resettling your baby. Over a few days you will ideally see that the time spent settling is reducing. Sometimes it is easy to forget how long you were spending and how the situation has improved. When you look at your progress you will realise how far you have come!

TIME OVER 24 HOURS

	6 AM	7 AM	8 AM	9 AM	10 AM	11 AM	12 MD	1 PM	2 PM	3 PM	4 PM	
0												
5												
10												
15												
20												
25												
30												
35												
40												
45												
50												
55												
60												
TOTAL												

MINUTES SPENT SETTLING

	5 PM	6 PM	7 PM	8 PM	9 PM	10 PM	11 PM	12 MN	1 AM	2 AM	3 AM	4 AM	5 AM

Settling progress chart

TIME OVER 24 HOURS

	6 AM	7 AM	8 AM	9 AM	10 AM	11 AM	12 MD	1 PM	2 PM	3 PM	4 PM	
0												
5												
10												
15												
20												
25												
30												
35												
40												
45												
50												
55												
60												
TOTAL												

MINUTES SPENT SETTLING

	5 PM	6 PM	7 PM	8 PM	9 PM	10 PM	11 PM	12 MN	1 AM	2 AM	3 AM	4 AM	5 AM

Settling progress chart

TIME OVER 24 HOURS

	6 AM	7 AM	8 AM	9 AM	10 AM	11 AM	12 MD	1 PM	2 PM	3 PM	4 PM	
0												
5												
10												
15												
20												
25												
30												
35												
40												
45												
50												
55												
60												
TOTAL												

MINUTES SPENT SETTLING

	5 PM	6 PM	7 PM	8 PM	9 PM	10 PM	11 PM	12 MN	1 AM	2 AM	3 AM	4 AM	5 AM

Settling progress chart

TIME OVER 24 HOURS

	6 AM	7 AM	8 AM	9 AM	10 AM	11 AM	12 MD	1 PM	2 PM	3 PM	4 PM	
0												
5												
10												
15												
20												
25												
30												
35												
40												
45												
50												
55												
60												
TOTAL												

MINUTES SPENT SETTLING

	5 PM	6 PM	7 PM	8 PM	9 PM	10 PM	11 PM	12 MN	1 AM	2 AM	3 AM	4 AM	5 AM

Personal notes

CHAPTER 5

Babies
6–12 months old

General sleep information	89
About crying	89
Signs of tiredness or 'tired cues'	91
Quiet wind down time	91
Settling your 6–12 month old	92
Modified Controlled Comforting	93
During the day	95
During the night	97
Looking after yourself	97
Points to remember	99
Frequently asked questions	100
Conclusion	104
Management plan	104
Personal notes	126

CHARTS

The Modified Controlled Comforting flow chart	96
Weekly feed, play, progress charts	110
Settling progress chart	118

General sleep information

From 6 to 12 months, babies are learning a great deal. They are becoming more aware of their environment and the people around them. They are also becoming more active and begin to sit, crawl and may even start to walk. As they become older they gradually need less sleep during the day and have longer periods of sleep overnight. Most babies between 6 and 12 months need 2–3 sleeps during the day.

To encourage babies of this age to sleep without waking overnight it is best to meet all their nutritional and social needs during the day. If your baby has been used to being fed to sleep they may wake overnight. They find that when they rouse between sleep cycles the breast or bottle that was there when they went to sleep has disappeared. Your baby may want to re-create this situation so that she can return to sleep. The only way that she can tell you this is by crying out.

Babies of this age usually respond well to a certain amount of predictability in their days. They learn to understand what to expect if a particular sequence or pattern is followed. A 'feed, play, sleep' pattern during the day will give you and your baby a pattern that is not unnecessarily rigid or too linked to time. To achieve this, look at all the activities that a baby of this age requires in her day.

Refer to Chapter 2 for more information about the 'feed, play, sleep' pattern and its benefits. An important part of this pattern is learning to become aware of the signs that your baby gives you to tell you that she is tired. It is sometimes easy to misread these signs.

It may also be helpful to view this time in your baby's development as a 'window of opportunity' in terms of altering her sleeping behaviour. It is probably going to be easier to alter behaviour at this stage of her life rather than when she is older. Although initially these techniques take effort and require consistency, they will get results.

About crying

Like adults, many babies find change occurring in their life disruptive or difficult. They probably won't understand what is happening if their feeding or sleeping patterns are altered. It is normal for your baby to cry to let you know that she doesn't understand. Gradually, as she begins to respond to the sleep messages and the settling techniques, the crying lessens and may cease.

During the settling process, babies often cry. Their cry usually builds up to a 'peak' before it quietens down again. When you put your baby into her cot her crying may begin with a 'grizzle' and then escalate until it becomes intense and loud. This is known as the 'crying peak'. Once babies reach this crying peak, they usually continue to cry but have intermittent periods of quiet. Some babies may begin to settle after their crying has peaked once.

It is often difficult for parents to listen to their baby crying. Many parents find their baby's cry too distressing to allow them to reach the crying peak. However, by supporting babies through this time and giving them clear sleep messages (rather than picking them up) they will learn to quieten and ultimately settle to sleep on their own.

The diagram shows the point at which the crying peaks. Parents often feel like they want to quit before this point is reached. The 'quitting point', when the cry is becoming more intense, is an indication that the cry will usually peak within about five minutes. This will be followed by shorter, less intense bouts of crying. Occasionally, but not always, a baby will build up to a crying peak again. The time taken from the beginning of crying to when a baby settles and is relaxed can vary enormously.

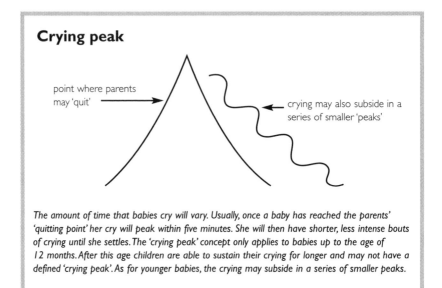

Crying peak

point where parents may 'quit' →

← crying may also subside in a series of smaller 'peaks'

The amount of time that babies cry will vary. Usually, once a baby has reached the parents' 'quitting point' her cry will peak within five minutes. She will then have shorter, less intense bouts of crying until she settles. The 'crying peak' concept only applies to babies up to the age of 12 months. After this age children are able to sustain their crying for longer and may not have a defined 'crying peak'. As for younger babies, the crying may subside in a series of smaller peaks.

Think of ways that you can remain calm but determined if you feel that you want to quit.

Try to think of the settling and crying from your baby's point of view. Picking her up when the crying is getting louder will not help her to learn to sleep. However, giving clear and consistent messages that you want her to go to sleep will help her through this learning process. Your baby may cry and protest while settling, but this is often less traumatic than being awake for hours on end and becoming overtired and grizzly. Try not to focus on the crying because it will stop. Focus on giving your baby clear sleep messages.

Signs of tiredness or 'tired cues'

It can be very difficult to understand the tired cues of babies who are poor sleepers or have disrupted sleeping patterns. Sometimes when your baby is tired she will give you signs like sucking her hands and/or crying. It can be easy to mistake these signs for hunger or perhaps interpret her behaviour as being bored or frustrated. Alternatively she can look wide awake! As she begins to sleep better it will become easier to recognise her tired signs.

Babies over 6 months of age may show some of the tired signs of younger babies such as yawning, grimacing or jerky movements. In addition the following tired signs may be seen:

◎ Becoming uninterested or bored with surroundings or toys
◎ Concentration span lessens
◎ Needing constant entertaining
◎ Grizzling becomes more intense
◎ Needing more physical contact
◎ Rubbing eyes, nose, ears, pulling hair
◎ Movements become less coordinated or she may become clumsy

Quiet wind down time

A consistent pattern that suits your baby and circumstances is an important place to start to help your child prepare for sleep. Aim to make this pattern simple and relaxing. Once a pattern is established and maintained, your baby will respond to being laid down for a sleep at home, and also at the homes of friends or relatives you visit. The sequence may vary for night and day sleeps, but needs to include a quiet wind down time. Quiet wind down time means decreasing stimulation and her activity. Remember, active busy babies respond best to settling strategies when they first show signs of tiredness. This may mean darkening the room and having a cuddle, gentle talking, reading a short story or singing a quiet song. If you have other children or a busy, noisy house, you may need to spend more time quietening your baby or you may involve the other child in a quiet story time.

However, if she starts to become more restless and whinge or cry, she may be getting overtired and it would be best to place her in the cot and commence settling.

Use the settling techniques for both day and night sleeps so that consistent messages are reinforced for your baby.

Settling your 6–12 month old

After a quiet time together, place your baby in her cot, on her back (see SIDS recommendations p. 26). Tuck her in and say something like 'Goodnight, have a good sleep'. It is important to give your baby the opportunity to settle herself. To do this, leave the room for a brief period of 30 seconds. Bedtime involves:

◎ Ensuring your baby is suitably dressed with a clean nappy.
◎ Darkening the room.
◎ Placing your baby in her cot and tucking her in. It is not appropriate to wrap a baby of this age. The startle reflex that can disturb young babies is no longer present. Many babies who have been wrapped when they are little will begin to wriggle and complain about being wrapped as they grow older. If your baby is used to being wrapped to settle it can take time to adjust to settling by being tucked in.
◎ Giving your baby the opportunity to settle herself.

Modified Controlled Comforting

Once in her bed, your baby may stay quiet and settle herself or she may grizzle and begin to cry. If, after 30 seconds, your baby continues to cry, return to the room and begin Modified Controlled Comforting.

Modified Controlled Comforting is a way to help a baby learn to establish an improved sleeping pattern. This includes settling themselves to sleep and resettling by themselves when they wake at the end of a sleep cycle either during the day or overnight. The process alternates 2–10 minutes of comforting with 2–10 minute periods of leaving the baby.

The principle behind the technique is that older babies are developmentally able to tolerate short periods of separation supported by periods of reassurance and comforting. Babies of this age are known to experience separation anxiety (being away from a parent), but they are developing a sense of 'object or person permanence'. This means they know that their parents still exist when they are not in the room with them. Modified Controlled Comforting was developed to reduce separation anxiety and to teach babies over 6 months to settle to sleep in the knowledge that they have developed this level of understanding. Also, from 6 months, babies are becoming more active, mobile and alert, so staying with them while they relax and settle can actually stimulate them further and may even make it more difficult for them to go to sleep.

To begin the sequence:

◎ Settle your baby in her cot on her back.
◎ Say goodnight and leave the room.
◎ Wait and listen for 30 seconds.
◎ If she cries, enter the room and commence settling techniques while she is on her back. If she does not respond you may need to turn your baby onto her side with her face away from you.

Spend only 2–10 minutes consoling and comforting your baby. She should be comforted in her cot with minimal stimulation. Start your settling with 'hands on' comforting, such as patting or stroking, as described on pp. 56–57. When using the settling techniques, observe your baby for her responses. Use only one or two strategies for the 2–10 minutes so that you do not confuse or stimulate her by using a number of techniques in a short period. Remember, it is important that she does not fall asleep while you are using the settling techniques so

PRE-SLEEP SIGNS

Use the settling techniques to quieten and relax your baby and watch for pre-sleep signs. When you see these, it is time to leave the room so that your baby can settle herself to sleep. These signs include:

- Becoming still and relaxed
- Loud crying has stopped
- Noises becoming more tuneful
- Eyelids becoming heavier and fluttering
- Slower, more rhythmic breathing
- A prolonged sigh
- Nestling into the mattress

watch for her pre-sleep signs (see box above). The aim is to teach her to go to sleep by herself. If she becomes quiet and relaxed, leave the room. If after 10 minutes your baby is still crying, leave the room.

- Leave her room and stay outside for **2 minutes**.

If she is crying, return to the room after the 2 minutes have passed and settle her using the settling techniques. Again, this may take between 2–10 minutes. If she becomes quiet and relaxed, leave the room. If after ten minutes your baby is still crying, leave the room.

- Leave her room and stay outside for **4 minutes**.

If she is still crying after the 4 minutes have elapsed, return to the room and settle her using the settling techniques. This may take between 2–10 minutes. If she becomes quiet and relaxed, leave the room. If after ten minutes your baby is still crying, leave the room.

◎ Leave the room and stay outside for **6 minutes**.

If she is crying after the 6 minutes have passed, return to the room and resettle her for between 2–10 minutes. If she becomes quiet and relaxed leave the room. If, after ten minutes, your baby is still crying leave the room.

◎ Leave the room and stay outside for **8 minutes**.

If she is crying after the 8 minutes have passed, return to the room and settle her for between 2–10 minutes. If she becomes quiet and relaxed leave the room. If after 10 minutes your baby is still crying, leave the room.

◎ Leave the room and stay outside for **10 minutes**.

If your baby is still awake and crying, continue to use settling techniques for between 2–10 minutes to quieten her then leave the room for 10-minute periods. Remember, leave the room when she becomes quiet.

You do not need to stay in with her for the whole 10 minutes each time. (Refer to the flow chart on the next page.)

Try to stay calm and relaxed. We will talk about ways that might help you to do this later.

If your baby is standing up when you are trying to settle her, gently lie her down, tuck her in and try to settle her with a supporting hand on her shoulder or hip.

It is not necessary to re-enter the room when all is quiet after the allotted time. Some parents may feel anxious about their baby at this point, particularly if the settling process has taken a while. Try to resist the temptation to go in and look straight away, because she may be quiet but not yet asleep or she could be in a light sleep and easily woken. This would undo all the hard work that you have both done.

Once your baby is soundly asleep, gently turn her onto her back. If she is on top of the bedclothes you could gently cover her with another blanket and tuck it in.

During the day

During the day, aim to persevere with Modified Controlled Comforting for up to 1 hour. If your baby has not settled by then, get her up and

Modified Controlled Comforting flow chart

For babies 6–12 months

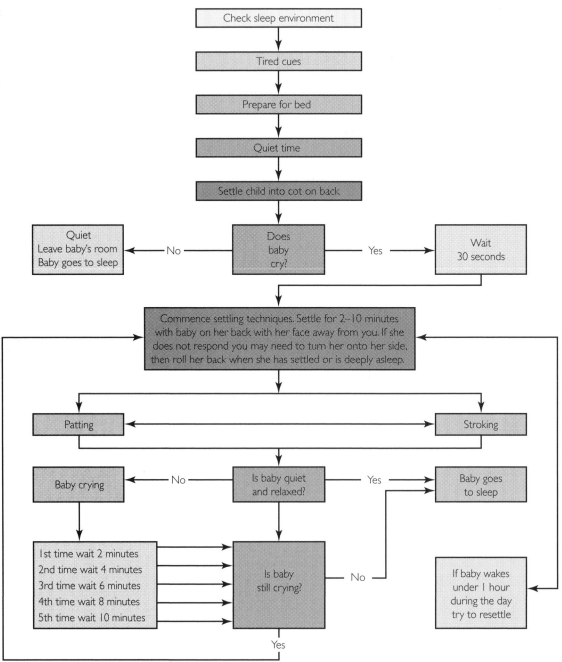

Note: *If you feel you are able, you can persist with these techniques for up to one hour. For resettling up to half an hour is recommended. At night time persist with the techniques until your baby settles.*

both of you can have a break. Give her a drink of water and a cuddle and let her have a play. Watch for her tired cues, then, when you are both ready, try again.

If your baby settles to sleep but sleeps for less than 1 hour, try to resettle her. A sleep of less than 1 hour will mean that she has only slept for 1 sleep cycle. The aim of the technique is to teach her to resettle herself if she wakes between sleep cycles. If you can, try Modified Controlled Comforting for another half-hour to resettle her.

During the night

If your baby is feeding well and having her nutritional needs met during the day and you have decided to gradually wean her off night feeds, try waking her for a late milk feed (e.g. 11 pm). You may then like to follow the settling strategies overnight after the late feed rather than feeding her when she wakes. When you and your baby are ready, you can gradually make this feed earlier until you are ready to replace it with settling only. If you are breastfeeding, remember to wean night feeds slowly and express for comfort if necessary to avoid mastitis.

The key to establishing an improved sleeping pattern is being consistent and persistent. If your baby wakes during the night, try to persevere with the Modified Controlled Comforting technique as long as you can. Continue Modified Controlled Comforting at 10-minute intervals. If, however, you find that you are becoming too upset, get your baby up for a brief cuddle or offer a small amount of water. Try to keep your baby in her own room with minimal lighting or stimulation. This will continue to give her consistent sleep messages and not 'awake' or 'playtime' messages.

Then, when you are ready, try again.

Looking after yourself

The following tips may make it easier for you to implement the Modified Controlled Comforting technique and enable you to follow through with your desire to alter your baby's sleeping patterns.

Minutes can seem like hours when you are listening to your baby crying. A watch with a second hand will help you know the exact time since you have settled her and left the room. A timer may also be helpful.

Keep pen and paper handy to record the number of times your baby wakes and how long she takes to settle. Charting may help to give you an idea of your progress. It will also reinforce the need for you to be consistent and to keep persevering with the strategies. Use the settling progress chart on p. 118.

The Modified Controlled Comforting technique can be very difficult if your baby is protesting loudly. Some parents worry about what others will think they might be doing to their baby. Discuss what is going on with the other members of your household and, if necessary, your neighbours.

◎ Be positive. It is hard work, but a worthwhile investment.
◎ Practise deep breathing exercises or relaxation techniques.
◎ Listen to music.
◎ Remind yourself that this is a small part of a big picture and you need to remember your long-term goals.
◎ Plan for support during the process. This may involve arrangements with a friend or family member to give you time out during the day or someone to be with you during the Modified Controlled Comforting period.
◎ Talk to someone about how you are feeling.
◎ Congratulate yourself and your baby on the small steps of progress that you make, not just the larger ones.
◎ Reward yourself for progress that you make and for hanging in there.

Like adults, babies are individuals and vary in their response to change. Experience has shown that a struggle to achieve a new pattern is rarely fruitless, so hang in there! Sometimes it may be really hard to keep going and you may need to take time out. You could modify the process but try to keep within the basic principles. You may decide to change the comforting timing or length of time waiting outside her room. For example, you may like to repeat the periods of time that you leave your child crying (2 minutes, 2 minutes; 4 minutes, 4 minutes, etc.) or decide that 6 rather than 10 minutes is the maximum time you will leave your child. It is important that changing her sleeping patterns is manageable for you but you need to recognise that modifying the process may result in slower progress. However, this may be preferable to giving up.

It is important, too, for all the family that you do not keep going if the process is too stressful or it is not okay for you. It may be necessary for your partner or a friend to take over. You may decide that the time is not right for change in your lives now or that you need more support to implement the strategies. None of these is a bad reflection on you but rather a positive acknowledgement of the importance of looking after yourself and being able to recognise your limits. This is far healthier than getting angry or punishing yourself or your baby. It is also important to reward both yourself and your baby. Tell her that she is making great progress and how proud you are of her. Don't forget to praise yourself as well!

Remember that you may have unexpected feelings regarding separation from your baby. You may have been used to holding and cuddling your baby for long periods of time in your efforts to get her to sleep. Think about something that you would like to do with the extra time that you will have when your baby is sleeping. Remember, too, that your baby will probably be happier when she is awake if she is getting adequate sleep so you may enjoy your time with her even more.

Points to remember

- ◎ Start the techniques when you know you can put other activities aside and focus on you and your baby.
- ◎ Start the techniques when you know you can see the program through.
- ◎ Start the program to help your baby establish an improved sleeping pattern when you are both well.
- ◎ Watch for early tired cues.
- ◎ A consistent pattern will help your baby prepare for sleep.
- ◎ Have a quiet wind down time with your baby before settling her in her cot.
- ◎ Place her in the cot awake.
- ◎ Use settling strategies to quieten only, not to put your baby to sleep.
- ◎ During the day, resettle her if she sleeps less than 1 hour.
- ◎ Be aware that you may have unexpected feelings regarding separation from your baby. Think about what you would like to do with the extra time you will have when she is sleeping.
- ◎ If there are times when your baby won't settle or resettle herself to sleep, don't feel bad or think that it has been a waste of time. The repetition of the settling techniques is valuable and she will eventually learn.

- The long term aim is for your baby to be able to settle and resettle herself.
- Babies of this age are able to tolerate periods of separation as long as they are not extensive and they are followed by reassurance.
- Focus on giving clear sleep messages, not on the crying, as the crying will stop.
- Take care of yourself.
- Remember: you can do it!

Frequently asked questions

During Modified Controlled Comforting my baby grizzles intermittently. What do you suggest?

If your baby is grizzling intermittently and you feel okay, leave her alone in her room. If this grizzling persists and she is not settling, re-enter the room and give quiet, clear sleep messages at 10-minute intervals. This may be enough for her to become quiet and relaxed. If she begins to cry, recommence Modified Controlled Comforting.

What do I do if my baby is quiet when I leave her room but starts to cry a few minutes later?

If your baby is quiet when you leave her room this is fine. Start your actual timing from when your baby begins to cry, then wait the allocated time until you re-enter her room. For example: you were due to wait 6 minutes outside her room but your baby was quiet for four minutes, before she started to cry. Therefore, wait 6 minutes from the point of time when your baby started crying before returning to the room.

Would a persistently crying baby settle better if left for longer than the ten minutes?

It is not recommended that you leave a baby crying by herself for any longer than 10 minutes as she may become more upset and harder to settle. You are trying to teach her to settle herself to sleep. Sleep messages and comforting will help her achieve this.

During the comforting time of 2–10 minutes of settling techniques, my baby does not respond and I feel that it is becoming a struggle. Do I keep going?

If you feel that it is becoming a struggle while you are using the settling techniques, leave the room. Wait the allocated period of time before re-entering the room and then try to use the settling techniques again. As she learns through repetition, this reinforcement of sleep messages and settling strategies will help her to learn.

Sometimes when I put my baby into her cot I hear her playing and talking to herself. What do I do?

If, after you have placed your baby in her cot, you hear her playing, wait 10 minutes then re-enter the room. Tuck her in again and say 'Good-night'. Aim to give clear messages that it is time for sleep, not play. If she continues to play, keep re-entering the room and give brief sleep messages at 10-minute intervals.

What do I do with my other children when I am settling my baby?

Explain to your other children what you are doing in terms they can understand. Try to occupy them, for example:

◎ Keep some special toys for them to play with during this time.
◎ Suggest they 'settle' a favourite doll.
◎ Ask another person to be with them.
◎ Tape their favourite television show and encourage them to watch it while settling your baby.
◎ Alternatively, they might like to listen to a music or story tape.

Once you have settled your baby, thank your other children for letting you settle her undisturbed and spend a few minutes with them. They will be more likely to help you in this way again.

Different strategies will work at different times and you will need to be creative and flexible.

I am returning to work and my baby is going to childcare. What will I do?

Discuss the changes that you are planning to make to your baby's settling and sleeping pattern with the childcare centre. Some centres will try to continue with the same strategies but many will find it difficult because of the number of babies that they are looking after. Continue using the techniques whenever you are with your baby. It may take a little longer for them to be effective but with consistency and patience you and your baby will benefit.

I am unsure how to lead a normal life while I am changing my baby's patterns. Do I need to stay at home until this has happened?

Aim to begin using the techniques when you have a few days at home and can follow through with your plan. If you do have to go out, try to arrange appointments when you think that your baby will be awake. If you need to be out for longer, organise appointments for only half a day instead of the whole day. Your baby will be able to sleep at home for some of the day. Your baby may be overtired when you get home and you may have to persevere with the techniques a little bit longer. If you are able to settle your baby when you are out, aim to follow through with the techniques you've been using at home. This will not always be possible so don't be too hard on yourself.

I think that my baby's dummy has become a sleep association but am unsure how to get rid of it.

There are three ways that you can work on this issue. How you choose to get rid of the dummy is entirely up to you and how you are feeling and your baby's response.

Firstly, if your baby has a dummy in her mouth all the time you can limit its use to bedtime only. Remember, however, that babies learn to talk by making noises and gurgling. They may also settle themselves to sleep while making these noises. A dummy can restrict this process.

The second way is to get rid of the dummy completely. Some parents choose to do this immediately and will take away the dummy and never offer it again.

You may prefer to take a third, more gradual, approach. This would mean that you don't offer your baby her dummy when she first goes to bed but you make her wait a few minutes into the settling until you give it to her. You could increase this time by a couple of minutes each time you settle her for her sleep. For example, the first time you could wait 2 minutes, the next time, 4, etc. until you find that she will settle without the dummy.

Every time I enter the room during settling my child is sitting or standing in her cot. What do I do?

Enter the room and in a calm voice tell your child to lie down and go to sleep. At the same time gently pat the mattress to reinforce what you are saying.

My baby keeps standing up when I am trying to settle her. I have tried holding her down but this doesn't work. What can I do?

Babies do not learn to relax by being forced to lie down or being patted or body rocked very firmly or quickly. Sometimes during the settling process your baby may not respond to the strategies you are using by settling quietly or quickly. You may observe her becoming more irritable and crying louder. Some parents may feel frustrated, angry or anxious during this time. Rather than persisting with settling, leave the room for a few minutes or the allocated time until you feel calmer. Alternatively, you could get her up, do something pleasant together, such as a walk, and use the techniques when she is tired again.

During sleep, my baby turns onto her tummy. Do I turn her onto her back?

Around the age of 6 months, babies start to roll in their sleep. If she rolls onto her tummy reposition her onto her back. If she rolls again, then leave her. Check again that the sleeping environment is safe. (See SIDS recommendations, p. 26, and address the factors that are within your control. You could also contact the SIDS Foundation for more information – see the Resources section, p. 173.)

What should I do beyond the 10-minute mark during the daytime?

During the daytime, if you have reached the 10-minute interval and your child has not settled we suggest that you continue to leave your child for 10-minute intervals. If she is still crying after 10 minutes, return to her room to comfort her (again, spend only 2–10 minutes) until she is quiet and relaxed, then leave the room. If she has not settled to sleep after 1 hour, enter her room, open the curtains, talk positively to her and pick her up. For night-time suggestions, see p. 97.

Conclusion

Parents who consistently use age-appropriate settling strategies will see an improvement in their baby's sleep pattern by the end of the first week. However, always keep in mind that it may take a little longer to see an even greater improvement. It can take time to change behaviour that has been occurring for a long time.

Often parents also see an improvement in other aspects of their baby's behaviour. This can include eating, playing and an improvement generally in their interactions with those around them.

You may find that your baby reverts to a disrupted sleeping pattern after a change or illness. Sometimes there is no reason for a change in sleeping behaviour. Generally your baby will respond very quickly to the settling techniques if you need to use them again. Remember, it is important to be persistent and consistent. It is hard work, but it will prove to be a positive investment of time and energy, and will help everyone to get a better night's sleep.

> I cannot even put into words the effect that doing the program has had on our lives as a family, except to say I feel so much better and confident as a mother and my husband is feeling more confident as a father too. My depression has lifted as a result of getting sleep and having a more settled happy baby. **SUSAN**

Management plan

The following questions may be useful to consider before you commence the settling techniques with your baby during the day or night. It can be difficult trying to negotiate with your partner/support person when you are both tired and stressed. If you are planning to implement changes it is important that you both agree with what you are going to do. You are more likely to succeed if you are consistent with the techniques and strategies discussed. If you decide to implement these changes by yourself you will still find the following questions helpful.

Think about the questions and write down some responses. There may be other questions that you would like to add that are important to you.

Sleeping environment

Where is your baby going to sleep during this process?

_____

_____

_____

Where are your other children going to sleep?

_____

_____

_____

If your baby uses a dummy

Are you going to limit the use of the dummy?

_____

_____

_____

Are you going to stop the use of the dummy immediately?

_____

_____

_____

How long are you going to wait until you give her the dummy?

_____

_____

_____

Feeding baby overnight

Are you planning to feed your baby overnight?

_____

_____

If you are going to stop a night feed, how are you going to do this?

_____

_____

_____

Settling

How long are you going to persist with the techniques?

_____

_____

_____

a) During the day?

_____

_____

_____

b) During the night?

_____

_____

_____

Who is going to be responsible for settling?

_____

_____

_____

a) During the day?

_____

_____

_____

b) During the night?

_____

_____

_____

At what time will this responsibility change?

_____

_____

_____

Who is going to look after your other children while you are settling your baby?

_____

_____

_____

Who is involved with your baby that you may need to talk to about the changes that you plan to make? (For example, childcare worker, friends, family, neighbours.)

_____

_____

_____

Looking after yourself

What strategies are you going to use to support you through the settling? (For example, earphones, music.)

_____

_____

_____

If you are feeling cross or frustrated what will you do or who can you talk to?

_____

_____

_____

Who will be there to give you a break if you need one?

_____

_____

_____

What can you do for yourself as a reward for the changes that you have made?

_____

_____

_____

Weekly feed, play, sleep chart

It is easy to feel that you are up all night with your baby, or that she is constantly feeding or crying. It may be helpful to have an accurate picture of your baby's feed, play and sleep pattern, so that you can maintain some perspective during stressful times. Completing this chart will also help you see the progress you are making with your baby. To fill in the chart, shade the area to show when your baby is asleep on each day. When your baby is awake, leave the spaces clear. When she has been fed, write an F in the box. Try to continue filling out the chart for 2–3 weeks. You will begin to see patterns in your baby's life.

	6 AM	7 AM	8 AM	9 AM	10 AM	11 AM	12 MD	1 PM	2 PM	3 PM	4 PM	
MONDAY												
TUESDAY												
WEDNESDAY												
THURSDAY												
FRIDAY												
SATURDAY												
SUNDAY												

- ■ DENOTES SLEEPING
- □ DENOTES AWAKE
- F DENOTES FEED

	5 PM	6 PM	7 PM	8 PM	9 PM	10 PM	11 PM	12 MN	1 AM	2 AM	3 AM	4 AM	5 AM

Weekly feed, play, sleep chart

	6 AM	7 AM	8 AM	9 AM	10 AM	11 AM	12 MD	1 PM	2 PM	3 PM	4 PM	
MONDAY												
TUESDAY												
WEDNESDAY												
THURSDAY												
FRIDAY												
SATURDAY												
SUNDAY												

■ DENOTES SLEEPING
□ DENOTES AWAKE
F DENOTES FEED

	5 PM	6 PM	7 PM	8 PM	9 PM	10 PM	11 PM	12 MN	1 AM	2 AM	3 AM	4 AM	5 AM

Weekly feed, play, sleep chart

	6 AM	7 AM	8 AM	9 AM	10 AM	11 AM	12 MD	1 PM	2 PM	3 PM	4 PM	
MONDAY												
TUESDAY												
WEDNESDAY												
THURSDAY												
FRIDAY												
SATURDAY												
SUNDAY												

■ DENOTES SLEEPING
☐ DENOTES AWAKE
F DENOTES FEED

	5 PM	6 PM	7 PM	8 PM	9 PM	10 PM	11 PM	12 MN	1 AM	2 AM	3 AM	4 AM	5 AM

Weekly feed, play, sleep chart

	6 AM	7 AM	8 AM	9 AM	10 AM	11 AM	12 MD	1 PM	2 PM	3 PM	4 PM	
MONDAY												
TUESDAY												
WEDNESDAY												
THURSDAY												
FRIDAY												
SATURDAY												
SUNDAY												

■ DENOTES SLEEPING
□ DENOTES AWAKE
F DENOTES FEED

	5 PM	6 PM	7 PM	8 PM	9 PM	10 PM	11 PM	12 MN	1 AM	2 AM	3 AM	4 AM	5 AM

Settling progress chart

When you fill in this chart over a 24-hour period, it will allow you to see how much time you are spending settling and resettling your baby. Over a few days you will ideally see that the time spent settling is reducing. Sometimes it is easy to forget how long you were spending and how the situation has improved. When you look at your progress you will realise how far you have come!

TIME OVER 24 HOURS

	6 AM	7 AM	8 AM	9 AM	10 AM	11 AM	12 MD	1 PM	2 PM	3 PM	4 PM	
0												
5												
10												
15												
20												
25												
30												
35												
40												
45												
50												
55												
60												
TOTAL												

MINUTES SPENT SETTLING

	5 PM	6 PM	7 PM	8 PM	9 PM	10 PM	11 PM	12 MN	1 AM	2 AM	3 AM	4 AM	5 AM

Settling progress chart

TIME OVER 24 HOURS

	6 AM	7 AM	8 AM	9 AM	10 AM	11 AM	12 MD	1 PM	2 PM	3 PM	4 PM	
0												
5												
10												
15												
20												
25												
30												
35												
40												
45												
50												
55												
60												
TOTAL												

MINUTES SPENT SETTLING

	5 PM	6 PM	7 PM	8 PM	9 PM	10 PM	11 PM	12 MN	1 AM	2 AM	3 AM	4 AM	5 AM

Settling progress chart

TIME OVER 24 HOURS

	6 AM	7 AM	8 AM	9 AM	10 AM	11 AM	12 MD	1 PM	2 PM	3 PM	4 PM	
0												
5												
10												
15												
20												
25												
30												
35												
40												
45												
50												
55												
60												
TOTAL												

MINUTES SPENT SETTLING

	5 PM	6 PM	7 PM	8 PM	9 PM	10 PM	11 PM	12 MN	1 AM	2 AM	3 AM	4 AM	5 AM

Settling progress chart

TIME OVER 24 HOURS

	6 AM	7 AM	8 AM	9 AM	10 AM	11 AM	12 MD	1 PM	2 PM	3 PM	4 PM	
0												
5												
10												
15												
20												
25												
30												
35												
40												
45												
50												
55												
60												
TOTAL												

MINUTES SPENT SETTLING

	5 PM	6 PM	7 PM	8 PM	9 PM	10 PM	11 PM	12 MN	1 AM	2 AM	3 AM	4 AM	5 AM

Personal notes

CHAPTER 6

Children
1–4 years old

General sleep information	129
Night feeds	129
About crying	130
Signs of tiredness	131
Quiet wind down time	131
Time for bed	132
Controlled Comforting	132
The gradual approach	135
Tricks of the trade	136
Looking after yourself	137
Points to remember	139
Frequently asked questions	140
Conclusion	143
Management plan	144
Personal notes	166

CHARTS

Controlled Comforting flow chart	134
Weekly eat, play, sleep chart	150
Comforting progress chart	158

General sleep information

Although the 'feed, play, sleep' pattern has been developed for babies, the same principles are relevant for children aged 1–4 who are still having two sleeps during the day. The term 'feed' for babies refers to a milk feed but for an older child this includes food and a drink. Usually, the number of meals is three, the same as for an adult, and there will be healthy snacks between meals. Many of these children will still have a sleep between each meal, with a long period of sleep overnight. As they approach 18–24 months, some children will cut out their morning or afternoon sleep and have a middle of the day sleep instead.

Night feeds

Children of this age can work out how much they need to eat during the day so if your child is still waking at night for food, then this is just from habit. Think about decreasing the number of night feeds gradually or cut them out altogether. This would depend on how many feeds she is having and how you are feeding her.

> Penny's [aged 15 months] daytime appetite is enormous now that the many bottles of milk she drank overnight has ceased!
>
> **MEREDITH**

If you are breastfeeding frequently overnight it would be better to reduce the feeds gradually so that your breasts do not become uncomfortable. If you feel that your child is thirsty or she says that she is thirsty, offer her a drink of water from a cup.

Some parents give their young child a bottle to help them settle in bed. Sometimes they will have another one or two overnight. However, children of this age can obtain their nutritional requirements during the day and should not need a bottle during the night. Having a bottle in bed can cause choking or dental caries from milk washing over the teeth. There is also the increased risk of ear infection as milk may flow through to the ear canal if the child is drinking while lying down. In addition, the child may develop a 'learned hunger' and wake each night feeling hungry.

Having a bottle to settle can also become a sleep association. If you feel that your child is hungry or thirsty, give her a drink of milk before the quiet wind down time so that she has finished it before going to bed (see p. 131). It is recommended to start weaning her to a cup from 12 months of age.

About crying

Like adults, many children find change occurring in their life disruptive or difficult. They may not understand what is happening if their patterns are altered. It is normal that your child will cry or yell to let you know that she doesn't like what is happening. As their verbal skills increase, you may find that your child will cry and yell in protest. Her crying may decrease. Gradually, as your child begins to respond to the sleep messages and the settling techniques that you are implementing, her behaviour will improve.

It is often difficult for parents to listen to their distressed child, and many parents find their child's behaviour too distressing to allow them to continue. But by supporting children through this time and giving them clear sleep messages they will learn to settle to sleep on their own.

Try to think of the settling and crying from your child's point of view. Picking her up or giving in when crying and yelling are getting louder will not help her to learn to sleep. However, giving clear and consistent messages that you want her to go to sleep will help her through this learning process. Your child may protest while settling, but this is often less traumatic than being awake for hours on end and being overtired and grizzly. Focus on giving her clear sleep messages. It will get better if you persevere.

> Ben [aged 2 years] is now sleeping through the night, having cut out all his night-time feeds. He now eats more than most other 2 year olds! It's great that we don't have him jumping into our bed all night. We feel like we have our life back and feel more confident in everything we do as parents. It's like a huge weight has been lifted from our shoulders!
>
> **ROBYN AND BRETT**

Signs of tiredness

When a child is tired or overtired her behaviour can become irritable, overactive or demanding. She may then find it difficult to relax at bedtime and struggle against going to sleep.

It is important to watch for your child's tired cues and settle her when the cues occur. Some examples of tired cues in 1–4 year olds are:

◎ Your child becomes more dependent. She needs to be near you and have you make decisions for her.
◎ She begins to whinge or cry.
◎ Her mood alternates between cheerful and tearful.
◎ She becomes increasingly clumsy and accident prone.
◎ She slows down or alternatively races around extra fast.
◎ She is fussy with food and drinks.
◎ She may rub her eyes, yawn, pull at her ears, perhaps pull her hair.
◎ Her behaviour may be indecisive.
◎ Some behaviour may be slightly aggressive.
◎ She may look for her 'security blanket' for comfort.

> We have learnt that consistency means every night for months, years perhaps. At least now we have a plan of attack rather than anarchy and anger. **JANE**

Quiet wind down time

Older children, just like babies, need to have a quiet wind down time before going to bed. As for babies, quiet wind down time means decreasing stimulation and reducing activities. This can include giving your child a cuddle, singing a gentle song, reading her a story, darkening the room to reduce stimulation, then placing her in bed.

It may only take a few minutes until she is relaxed but if your household is busy or noisy you may need to spend more time quietening your child.

By this age, your child may have chosen a blanket, piece of material or soft toy as a comfort. The importance of this 'transitional object' is that she has chosen it. Hence it will play a vital role in her wind down time.

Time for bed

If bedtime is a pleasant time, you and your child will both look forward to it. Aim to follow a pattern as consistently as you can.

A good place to start to help your child establish an improved sleep pattern is by developing a sequence of cues. By their repetition each night, these will signal to the child that bedtime is approaching. The following sequence of activities is a guideline for an evening pattern for young children:

- Dinner
- Bath time
- Drink of milk
- Cleaning teeth
- Clean nappy or take your child to the toilet
- Gentle singing, cuddles, reading stories
- Settle child for the night and tuck in the bedclothes
- Favourite soft toy to cuddle in bed
- Talk quietly (some children like their heads to be stroked)
- Say goodnight
- Leave her room promptly

At this point your child may settle herself to sleep, grizzle, cry or even yell.

Controlled Comforting

Young children need to learn how to go to sleep by themselves. If this is a new concept for them, they may need their parents' help. One very successful way of helping your child to learn to go to sleep is to use the technique called Controlled Comforting. This technique is based on an understanding of the developmental stage of a child over the age of 12 months. By this age, children have developed 'object and person permanence'. This means that they understand that even though an object or person has disappeared from view, they have not ceased to exist. They can therefore be left for longer intervals between parent comforting, knowing that you will return. This technique is not appropriate for young babies.

Controlled Comforting does not give the child a feeling of being abandoned, nor does it give her your presence 24 hours a day. It will result in your child, and therefore you and your family, obtaining a good night's sleep regularly. Before you start, it is helpful to have a brief talk with your child about what is going to happen at bedtime.

Your young child has been settled, using a similar pattern to that outlined in 'Time for bed'. If she begins to cry or protest:

◎ Leave the room. Check your watch. Leave her to cry for 2 minutes.
◎ If she is still crying after 2 minutes have elapsed, go back in saying, 'Goodnight, it's time for sleep'. Briefly reassure her for 30 seconds to 1 minute. Leave promptly.
◎ Check your watch. Leave her for 2 minutes longer than the last time; that is, 4 minutes.
◎ Repeat steps 1 and 2, increasing the time that you leave her alone for by an extra 2 minutes each time and progress as necessary to a total of 10 minutes: For example: 4 + 2 (6 minutes) then 6 + 2 (8 minutes) then 8 + 2 (10 minutes).

Do not leave your upset child for more than 10 minutes. By returning at 10-minute intervals you and your child will feel reassured and the sleep message is reinforced. Hopefully she will find her parents boring, as each time you re-enter, it is only for a brief period of 30 seconds to 1 minute. It can be hard not to respond to her crying but try to switch off your emotions – act like a robot and avoid eye contact with her. The aim is to give her very clear sleep messages and let her know that you are not there for entertainment or to engage in a long settling period. Try changing your tone of voice and let her know that you are serious. It is important not to get angry. Remember, these techniques do not teach your child to go to sleep by ignoring her protests completely or by scolding her.

It is not necessary to re-enter the room when all is quiet after the allotted time. Some parents may feel anxious about their child at this point, particularly if the settling process has taken a while. Try to resist the temptation to go in and look straight away, because she may be quiet but not yet asleep or she could be in a light sleep and easily woken. This would undo all the hard work that you have both done.

Controlled Comforting flow chart
For children over 1 year old

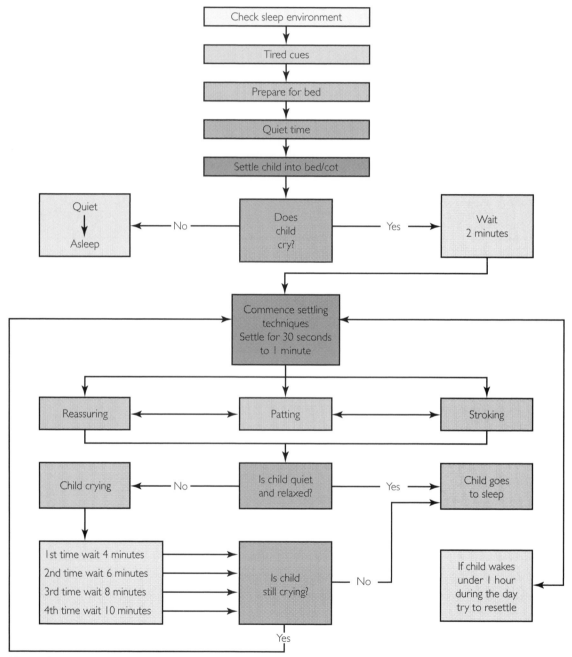

Note: *During the day you can persist with these techniques for up to one hour. For resettling up to half an hour is recommended. At night persist with the techniques until your child settles.*

If you feel you need to look, wait at least 10 to 15 minutes. If she is on top of the bedclothes you could gently cover her with another blanket and tuck it in. Remember, the aim is for you to help your child learn how to go to sleep by herself. If you stay with her until she drifts off to sleep she may expect you to do this every time she wakes. It is important that the sleep messages you give your child are very clear. The Controlled Comforting technique ensures that your child knows you are taking care of her, but that you are not available for play or conversation. Persevere with the technique; it is worthwhile continuing.

Provided you feel that you are coping, persist with the Controlled Comforting for up to 1 hour during the day. If trying to resettle your child you could try for up to half an hour.

Day or night, if you find that you are too distressed to continue, it is okay to stop and comfort your child and start again next sleep time. Success takes time, persistence and consistency. If at first your child does not respond, don't give up and feel it does not work. Remember, your child is changing a pattern she may have known for many months or perhaps all her life. She will master this new skill with your patient, consistent teaching and support.

The gradual approach

Some parents prefer to work more gradually on their child's sleeping difficulty, especially if they have spent time lying down next to their child to settle her. The following approach will be effective but, as with any behaviour change, will take time and require you to be consistent and persistent in your approach.

Ensure your child has a pleasant bedtime pattern.

Explain to her that you will sit on a chair beside the bed until she falls asleep. Tell her: 'If you stay in the bed, I will stay in the room and the door will stay open. If you get out of bed I will leave the room and close the door.' You may like to put your hand on her to reassure her. However, avoid engaging in conversation or games.

If she climbs out of bed return her to bed. Tell her in a firm voice, 'You need to stay in bed, otherwise I will have to leave the room and close the door'.

If she climbs out of bed again, return her to bed. Tell her in a firm voice, 'You need to stay in bed. I will leave the room and close the door the next time you get out of bed'.

If she climbs out of bed again return her to bed. Tell her in a firm voice, 'You have got out of bed, so now I am going to leave the room and close the door'. Commence controlled comforting.

After the allocated time out of the room, for example, 2 minutes, go back into her room, put her back in bed if necessary and return to your chair. If she continues to gets out of bed, continue the controlled comforting process.

Provided she stays in bed, sit on the chair until she falls asleep.

Each sleep time, move the chair a little way further from your child's bed.

Eventually, your aim will be to move the chair outside the bedroom door as she will have learnt to settle herself to sleep. If your child persists in getting out of bed, see Frequently asked questions, p. 141, for more ideas.

> Now there are more smiles, kisses and hugs to share with Adam [aged 3 years]. We are all much happier now that we are getting enough sleep and some time for each other.
>
> **STEVE AND VOULA**

Tricks of the trade

The following ideas may be helpful:

- ◎ The 'No choice' choice: Don't ask your child if she wants to go to bed. Let her know she will be going to bed shortly but do not argue with her about the time. Instead, allow her to make a choice of a different kind. For example, you might ask her to choose a story for you to read to her before bed. (Agree on the number of stories you are going to read however!)
- ◎ Avoid lively play before bedtime as this can result in the child being overstimulated and contribute to overtiredness.
- ◎ Before you settle your child to bed play a quiet sleep game. For example, let your child put her favourite teddy or favourite toy to sleep, then it will be her turn to go to bed.
- ◎ Tell your child that after her sleep, she'll be able to do a fun activity.

For example, 'When you wake up from your sleep, we will go to the park'. Make sure that you follow through with the activity.

◎ Give your child positive praise for desired behaviour, so she feels loved and secure.

◎ For a 3 year old, you could also use a star chart, surprise box or dot-to-dot to encourage positive behaviour. (If you are unsure about these strategies speak to your health care professional.)

Looking after yourself

You will need to discuss the changes that you intend to make with other members of your household or family. This will help them to understand the changes and how you intend to implement them. They are then included and are able to support and participate in your effort.

Write down a management plan (see p 144). This can help you to be clear about what your aims are and the strategies you will use. In the middle of the night it is much easier to read a plan you have prepared beforehand, than try to locate the appropriate section in a book. If you and your partner are both going to share responsibility for introducing the technique make sure that you each understand what your roles will be. It is important to discuss this during the day, not in the middle of the night!

Use a watch with a second hand to time your stays with your child and to time the period that you stay outside the room. The watch helps you to know the exact time you left the room. When your child is crying, whether night or day, time can often seem to pass more slowly than it really does.

At night, the Controlled Comforting technique can be very difficult to use if your child is protesting loudly. Some parents worry about what other people will think that they might be doing to their child. As well as discussing what is going on with the other members of your household (as suggested earlier), you might consider discussing it with your neighbours.

Use a progress chart (on p. 158 at the end of this chapter). This will give you an idea of your child's progress, and reinforce the need for you to be consistent and persistent with the techniques. By keeping a chart for each day and night you will be able to see improvement in her sleep patterns and be inspired to continue. Shade in the times that your child

> I have used these techniques and it has been an amazing transformation. Emma [aged 3 years] now puts herself to sleep night and day. I had to persist but the results have been worth it. Sometimes I think we have a different child now!
>
> JANINE

is asleep. For example, if she has slept from 1 pm to 3 pm, shade that whole area. You may also want to indicate the time spent awake and playing. When you put your child to bed, make sure you note the time. If you put her to bed at 8 pm and you spend 40 minutes using the Controlled Comforting technique, indicate this on the chart with hatching, or shading of a different colour.

Finally, remember to:

◎ Be positive about the process
◎ Reward yourself, even for the smallest success
◎ Listen to music
◎ Practise deep breathing exercises or relaxation techniques

Like adults, children are individuals and vary in their response to change. Experience has shown that a struggle to achieve a new pattern is rarely fruitless, so hang in there! On particular nights it may be really hard to keep going and you may need to take time out. You could modify the process but try to keep within the basic principles. You may decide to change the comforting timing or length of time waiting outside her room. For example, you may like to repeat the periods of time that you leave your child crying (2 minutes, 2 minutes; 4 minutes, 4 minutes, etc.) or decide that 6 rather than 10 minutes is the maximum time you will leave your child. It is important that changing your child's sleeping patterns is manageable for you but you, need to recognise that modifying the process may result in slower progress. However, this may be preferable to giving up.

It is important for all the family that you do not keep going if the process is too stressful or it is not okay for you. It may be necessary for your partner or a friend to take over. You may decide that the time is not right for change in your lives or that you need more support to implement the strategies. None of these is a bad reflection on you but rather a positive acknowledgement of the importance of looking after yourself and being able to recognise your limits. This is far healthier than getting angry or punishing yourself or your child. It is also important to reward both yourself and your young child. Tell her that you are making great progress and how proud you are of her. Don't forget to also tell yourself!

Be aware that you may have unexpected feelings regarding separation from your child. You may have been used to holding and cuddling your child for long periods of time in your efforts to get her to sleep. Think about something that you would like to do with the extra time that you will have when your child is sleeping. Remember, too, that your child will probably be happier when she is awake if she is getting adequate sleep so you may enjoy your time with her even more.

Points to remember

◎ Start the technique when you know you can put other activities aside and focus on you and your child, and when you know you can see it through.

◎ Help your child establish an improved sleeping pattern when she is well.

◎ Watch for tired cues.

◎ Establish a consistent pattern to help your child prepare for bed.

◎ Have a quiet wind down time before bed.

◎ Place your child into bed awake.

◎ During the day, resettle your child if she sleeps for less than 1 hour.

◎ Be aware that you may have unexpected feelings regarding separation from your child. Think about what you might like to do with the extra time that you will have while your child is sleeping.

◎ The long term aim is for your child to be able to settle and resettle herself to sleep.

◎ Focus on giving clear sleep messages, not on the crying or yelling as it will stop.

◎ Take care of yourself.

◎ Remember: you can do it!

Frequently asked questions

I am returning to work and my child is going to childcare. What will I do?

It is important to discuss the changes that you are planning to make to your child's settling and sleeping pattern with the childcare centre. Some centres will try to continue with the same strategies but many will find it difficult because of the number of children that they are looking after.

Continue using the techniques whenever you are with your child. The techniques will work more effectively and quickly if you can use them for a couple of days without interruption. You could begin using them on the weekend if your child is in childcare every weekday. It may take a little longer for them to be effective but with consistency and patience you and your child will benefit.

I am unsure how to lead a normal life while I am changing my child's patterns. Do I need to stay at home until this has happened?

Aim to begin using the techniques when you have a few days at home and can follow through with your plan. If you do have to go out, try to arrange appointments when you think that your child will be awake. If you need to be out for longer, organise appointments for only half a day instead of the whole day so that your child will be able to sleep at home. Your child may be overtired when you get home and you may have to persevere with the techniques a little bit longer. If you are able to settle your child when you are out, aim to follow through with the techniques you've been using at home. This will not always be possible so don't be too hard on yourself.

During daytime settling my child continually talks to herself or gets up to play with her toys. What do you suggest?

If she does not go to sleep and is not distressed, you may choose to leave her in her room for an hour or a bit longer to have a rest by herself, this is dependent on her age. Being able to play independently and amuse themself is an important part of a child's development. Enjoy it!

However, if the need for sleep is great and your child continues to play, you will need to go into her room at 10-minute intervals and give her clear sleep messages.

Every time I enter the room during settling my child is sitting or standing in her cot. What do I do?

Enter the room and in a calm voice tell your child to lie down and go to sleep. At the same time gently pat the mattress to reinforce what you are saying.

What do I do if my child always climbs out of bed and follows me out of the room?

a) Return your child to her bed. Tell her in a firm voice what the bedtime rules are: 'You need to stay in bed and I will leave the door open. If you get out of bed I will close the door'. Leave the room. Then:

b) If she climbs out and follows you out of the room again, return your child to her bed and tell her in a firm voice: 'You have got out of your bed so now I am going to close the door'. Close the door.

c) If when the door is closed she climbs out of bed and bangs on the door, wait the prescribed time of the Controlled Comforting, for example, 2 minutes. Return her to the bed by walking with her, not carrying or cuddling her and repeat the above techniques, increasing the delay time as in Controlled Comforting (see p. 132). Remember, this is a short term strategy – if you are calm and consistent children learn quickly. If she stays in bed, leave the door ajar.

You may need to set limits in conjunction with Controlled Comforting. Explain the rules to your child, including the consequences. This helps her learn what is expected of her and how she should behave. If she doesn't stay in bed it's important that you follow through with realistic consequences.

Your child may go to sleep on the floor of her bedroom. If it is during the day, make sure that she is safe and warm. However if this happens at night you may wake her and quietly walk her back to bed.

What do I do if my child vomits when I am trying to settle her?

Some children unintentionally learn that they receive attention if they vomit. It is important that you continue to give them clear sleep messages at this time. Do not punish your child if she vomits, but behave calmly and clean her up in the room. Try not to over-comfort her and then recommence Controlled Comforting. To reduce the possibility of vomiting, separate the feeding and drinking time from bedtime by

30 minutes. This will mean that your child has digested her food and drink.

While I'm settling my child, she continually turns on the light. What do I do?

Remove the light globe or lamp. If a child learns to stay in bed with the door open she has access to filtered light.

My child keeps calling out 'I need a drink'. Do I give her one?

Take a small drink of water only into the room. This is to be drunk immediately and then removed.

My child always calls out 'I need to go to the toilet' or 'I have a dirty nappy'. What do you suggest?

Change the nappy in the cot or bed to avoid reinforcing the behaviour but do not punish her. If she needs to go to the toilet, walk her there directly and return her immediately to her room. Aim not to over-attend or give any cuddles to her at this time. Recommence Controlled Comforting straight away.

I think that my child's dummy has become a sleep association but am unsure how to get rid of it.

There are three ways that you can work on this issue.

Firstly, if your child has a dummy in her mouth all the time you can limit its use to bedtime only. Remember, however, that children learn to talk by making noises. They may also settle themselves to sleep while making these noises. A dummy can restrict this process.

The second method is to get rid of the dummy completely. Some parents choose to do this immediately and will take away the dummy and never offer it again.

Thirdly, some parents prefer to take a more gradual approach for children. This would mean that you don't offer your child her dummy when she first goes to bed, making her wait a few minutes into the settling until you give it to her. You could increase this time by a couple of minutes each time you settle her for her sleep. For example, the first time you could wait two minutes, the next, four, and so on until you find that she will settle without the dummy. Parents could introduce a star chart if their child is aged 3 or over. The star chart enables the child to participate in saying goodbye to her dummy and gain recognition for her efforts.

I find that the lead-up to bedtime takes longer and longer and my child asks for more and more stories. What do you suggest?

You and your child can select the number of stories together, but once this is agreed, stick to it despite the tears.

My child is crying through the night. Could it be nightmares?

Nightmares are quite common for young children, especially between the ages of 3 and 5. They mostly occur towards morning: the child wakes, can tell vivid details and responds to comforting. Triggers may be an exciting event, scary stories or television. A relaxing bedtime routine can avoid this. Do not check for monsters: the child may think they are real. Night terrors are less common. They happen earlier in the night, the child does not fully wake and may be inconsolable. Although distressing for parents, the child will have no recollection of the event the next morning. Do not try to wake your child, but offer comfort if she asks for help.

My 15 month old has started to climb out of her cot.

This now becomes a safety issue. You have two options to consider: think about placing a mattress on the floor until she is able to climb into a bed; alternatively you could leave the cot side down to let her climb out safely. In both situations, think about what is in her room and remember to create a safe environment.

Conclusion

Parents who consistently use age-appropriate settling strategies will see a noticeable improvement in their child's sleep pattern by the end of the first week. However, always keep in mind that it may take a little longer to see an even greater improvement. This can sometimes take up to three weeks. It can take time to change behaviour that has been occurring for a long while.

Life is pure bliss! Hannah [aged 15 months] now sleeps 10–12 hours per night and has two 2-hour sleeps during the day. We are now enjoying every waking moment with her. SAM

Often parents will see an improvement in other aspects of their child's behaviour. This can include eating, playing and generally in their interactions with those around them.

You may find that your child reverts to a disrupted sleeping pattern after a change or illness occurs. Sometimes there is no reason for a change in sleeping behaviour. Generally your child will respond very quickly to the settling techniques if you need to use them again.

The settling strategies discussed have proved to be very effective; however success is dependent upon your consistency and motivation.

It is hard work, but it will prove to be a positive investment of time and energy, and will help everyone to get a better night's sleep.

Management plan

The following questions may be useful to consider before you commence the settling strategies with your young child during the day or night. It can be difficult trying to negotiate with your partner/support person when you are both tired and stressed during the middle of the night. If you are planning to implement changes it is important that you both agree with what you are going to do. You are more likely to succeed if you are consistent with the strategies discussed. If you decide to implement these changes by yourself you will still find the following questions helpful.

Think about the questions and write down some responses. There may be other questions that you would like to add that are important to you.

Sleeping environment

Where is your child going to sleep during this process?

_____

_____

_____

Where are your other children going to sleep?

_____

_____

_____

_____

Is your young child moving into a cot or a bed soon?

_____

_____

_____

_____

If your child uses a dummy

Are you going to limit the use of a dummy?

_____

_____

_____

_____

How long are you going to wait until you give her the dummy?

_____

_____

_____

Are you going to stop the use of the dummy immediately?

_____

_____

_____

Feeding your child overnight

Ceasing overnight feeds: how are you going to do this?

_____

_____

_____

_____

Settling

How long are you going to persist with the techniques?

_____

_____

_____

a) During the day?

_____

_____

_____

b) During the night?

_____

_____

_____

Who is going to be responsible for settling?

_____

_____

_____

_____

a) During the day?

_____

_____

_____

_____

b) During the night?

_____

_____

_____

_____

At what time will this responsibility change?

_____

_____

_____

_____

Who is going to look after your other children while you are settling your young child?

_____

_____

_____

Who is involved with your child that you may need to talk to about the changes that you plan to make? (For example, childcare worker, friends, family, neighbours.)

_____

_____

_____

Looking after yourself

What strategies are you going to use to support you through the settling? (For example, earphones.)

_____

_____

_____

If you are feeling cross or frustrated what will you do or who can you talk to?

_____

_____

_____

_____

Who will be there to give you a break if you need one?

_____

_____

_____

What can you do for yourself as a reward for the changes that you
have made?

_____

_____

_____

Weekly eat, play, sleep chart

It is easy to feel that you are up all night with your child, or that she is constantly eating or crying. It may be helpful to have an accurate picture of your child's eating/drinking, waking and sleeping pattern, so that you can maintain some perspective during stressful times. Completing this chart will also help you see the progress you are making with your child. To fill in the chart, shade the area to show when your child is asleep each day. When she is awake, leave the spaces clear. When she has eaten, write an M in the box. When she is playing write a P in the box. You will begin to see patterns in your child's life.

	6 AM	7 AM	8 AM	9 AM	10 AM	11 AM	12 MD	1 PM	2 PM	3 PM	4 PM	
MONDAY												
TUESDAY												
WEDNESDAY												
THURSDAY												
FRIDAY												
SATURDAY												
SUNDAY												

■ DENOTES SLEEPING
□ DENOTES AWAKE
F DENOTES FEED

	5 PM	6 PM	7 PM	8 PM	9 PM	10 PM	11 PM	12 MN	1 AM	2 AM	3 AM	4 AM	5 AM

Weekly eat, play, sleep chart

	6 AM	7 AM	8 AM	9 AM	10 AM	11 AM	12 MD	1 PM	2 PM	3 PM	4 PM	
MONDAY												
TUESDAY												
WEDNESDAY												
THURSDAY												
FRIDAY												
SATURDAY												
SUNDAY												

■ DENOTES SLEEPING
☐ DENOTES AWAKE
F DENOTES FEED

	5 PM	6 PM	7 PM	8 PM	9 PM	10 PM	11 PM	12 MN	1 AM	2 AM	3 AM	4 AM	5 AM

Weekly eat, play, sleep chart

	6 AM	7 AM	8 AM	9 AM	10 AM	11 AM	12 MD	1 PM	2 PM	3 PM	4 PM	
MONDAY												
TUESDAY												
WEDNESDAY												
THURSDAY												
FRIDAY												
SATURDAY												
SUNDAY												

■ DENOTES SLEEPING
☐ DENOTES AWAKE
F DENOTES FEED

	5 PM	6 PM	7 PM	8 PM	9 PM	10 PM	11 PM	12 MN	1 AM	2 AM	3 AM	4 AM	5 AM

Weekly eat, play, sleep chart

	6 AM	7 AM	8 AM	9 AM	10 AM	11 AM	12 MD	1 PM	2 PM	3 PM	4 PM	
MONDAY												
TUESDAY												
WEDNESDAY												
THURSDAY												
FRIDAY												
SATURDAY												
SUNDAY												

■ DENOTES SLEEPING
☐ DENOTES AWAKE
F DENOTES FEED

	5 PM	6 PM	7 PM	8 PM	9 PM	10 PM	11 PM	12 MN	1 AM	2 AM	3 AM	4 AM	5 AM

Comforting progress chart

When you fill in this chart over a 24-hour period, it will allow you to see how much time you are spending settling and resettling your child. Over a few days you will ideally see that the time spent settling is reducing. Sometimes it is easy to forget how long you were spending and how the situation has improved. When you look at your progress you will realise how far you have come!

TIME OVER 24 HOURS

	6 AM	7 AM	8 AM	9 AM	10 AM	11 AM	12 MD	1 PM	2 PM	3 PM	4 PM	
0												
5												
10												
15												
20												
25												
30												
35												
40												
45												
50												
55												
60												
TOTAL												

MINUTES SPENT SETTLING

	5 PM	6 PM	7 PM	8 PM	9 PM	10 PM	11 PM	12 MN	1 AM	2 AM	3 AM	4 AM	5 AM

Comforting progress chart

TIME OVER 24 HOURS

	6 AM	7 AM	8 AM	9 AM	10 AM	11 AM	12 MD	1 PM	2 PM	3 PM	4 PM	
0												
5												
10												
15												
20												
25												
30												
35												
40												
45												
50												
55												
60												
TOTAL												

MINUTES SPENT SETTLING

	5 PM	6 PM	7 PM	8 PM	9 PM	10 PM	11 PM	12 MN	1 AM	2 AM	3 AM	4 AM	5 AM

Comforting progress chart

TIME OVER 24 HOURS

	6 AM	7 AM	8 AM	9 AM	10 AM	11 AM	12 MD	1 PM	2 PM	3 PM	4 PM	
0												
5												
10												
15												
20												
25												
30												
35												
40												
45												
50												
55												
60												
TOTAL												

MINUTES SPENT SETTLING

	5 PM	6 PM	7 PM	8 PM	9 PM	10 PM	11 PM	12 MN	1 AM	2 AM	3 AM	4 AM	5 AM

Comforting progress chart

TIME OVER 24 HOURS

	6 AM	7 AM	8 AM	9 AM	10 AM	11 AM	12 MD	1 PM	2 PM	3 PM	4 PM	
0												
5												
10												
15												
20												
25												
30												
35												
40												
45												
50												
55												
60												
TOTAL												

MINUTES SPENT SETTLING

	5 PM	6 PM	7 PM	8 PM	9 PM	10 PM	11 PM	12 MN	1 AM	2 AM	3 AM	4 AM	5 AM

Personal notes

_____

_____

_____

_____

_____

_____

_____

_____

_____

_____

_____

_____

_____

_____

_____

_____

CHAPTER 7

Multiple births

More than one	169
Points to remember	169

More than one

There is a big difference between having just the one baby, and having two or more babies at the same time. Caring for more than one child is very physically and emotionally tiring, particularly in the first three years. Don't forget to look after yourself, and develop and use the supports that are around you.

Many parents find it useful to have their babies' feeding, waking and sleeping patterns synchronised. To achieve this, some established patterns may require change and the use of different strategies. This can create dilemmas, especially if one baby is already established in the patterns you want and you are concerned that any changes you make will adversely affect her 'settled' behaviour. It is common and normal for the 'settled' baby to become the 'unsettled' baby and vice versa, as children's behaviours and responses do change as they progress through developmental stages. It also helps for parents to recognise each child's unique personality, temperament and needs, and adjust their expectations accordingly.

The principles and strategies for achieving more settled patterns with twins or triplets are the same as previously discussed in this book. Refer to the chapter which contains the strategies for your babies' or children's age.

Points to remember

◎ With persistence and consistency you will achieve your goals.
◎ At first you might place both babies in the same cot. Remember the SIDS guidelines (see p. 26) and sleep each baby so that their feet are touching the end of the cot. When they start to disturb each other, it is time to move them into separate cots.
◎ Decide whether you want to put your babies/children in the same or separate bedrooms. In some instances, children settled in the same room can disturb each other, however this does not always happen, particularly in the long term. If children are in the same room they can be settled at the same time.
◎ Arrange cots to allow you to have physical contact with both babies/children at the same time during settling. For example, place cots close to each other so you can sit between them.

- Arrange feed times to coincide. This encourages shared play and settling times, and means you don't end up feeding constantly and can have a break.
- Reward and congratulate yourself for any progress you make.
- Joining a multiple birth club will provide the benefit of peer group support and is a great way to learn new tips and ways of managing more than one baby.

About Tweddle Child + Family Health Service

Tweddle Child + Family Health Service, located in the Melbourne suburb of Footscray, was established in 1920. Since that time, the service has been committed to supporting families with young children, from newborn to 4 years of age. Over the years Tweddle has operated in a number of different ways, redeveloping, expanding and implementing new services to meet changing community needs and expectations. The one theme that has remained constant over this time is the aim to strengthen the confidence of parents enabling them to nurture their young children and enjoy family life. Families experiencing difficulties with feeding, settling and sleep, a child's behaviour, family stress and conflict, and mild to moderate postnatal depression are all assisted through Tweddle's programs. Today, Tweddle offers its specialist expertise through a range of services including:

◎ Education: seminars and workshops are conducted at Tweddle and in the community for parents and professionals on many issues relating to family life. The seminars on settling and sleep management for families with young children are very popular and have assisted many parents.

◎ Professional consultancy and education: on the diverse range of difficulties that parents with young children can experience, including settling and sleep management, breastfeeding and understanding and managing their child's behaviour.

◎ Community day-stay programs: for parents experiencing difficulties with children from newborn to 4 years of age. Families attend a one day program during which they receive intensive support and assistance from Family Nurse Practitioners to address their particular difficulties.

◎ Family residential programs: for parents with children aged newborn to 4 years of age. Families are admitted to Tweddle for a number of nights and, with the expert help and support of Family Nurse Practitioners, address their family's particular difficulties.

◎ Research: on issues and difficulties experienced by families with young children.

Please call Tweddle on (03) 9689 1577 for further information.

List of resources

AUSTRALIAN CAPITAL TERRITORY

Australian Breastfeeding Association (ABA)
The ABA provides a 24-hour help line for parents requiring assistance with breastfeeding issues. Educational information on breastfeeding is also available.
Tel: (02) 6258 8928
Website: www.breastfeeding.asn.au

Australian Multiple Birth Association (AMBA)
The AMBA provides information and education, and counselling and support for mothers of multiple births. For your nearest contact call the national office:
Tel: (02) 9875 2404
Website: www.amba.org.au

Women's Centre for Health Matters
Tel: (02) 6290 2166
Health Info Line: (02) 6286 2043

Women's Health Service
Tel: (02) 6205 1078

Canberra Hospital
Yamba Drive
Garran ACT 2605
Tel: (02) 6244 2222
Website: www.canberrahospital.act.gov.au

ACT Community Health
You can contact ACT Community Health for information on all child health services provided in the ACT.
Tel: (02) 6207 9977

Women's Information and Referral Centre
Tel: (02) 6205 1075
Website: www.wirc.act.gov.au

ParentLine
9am–9pm, Mon–Fri
Tel: (02) 6287 3833

Lifeline
Tel: 131 114
Website: www.act.lifeline.org.au

Relationships Australia, ACT
Relationships Australia is an organisation that offers resources to couples, individuals and families to help enhance and support relationships. By phoning the free number below, your call will automatically be directed to the nearest Relationships Australia office in your area.
Toll-free: 1300 364 277
Website: www.relationships.com.au

Queen Elizabeth II Family Centre
Provides postnatal advice and assistance, as well as day stay and residential programs.
Tel: (02) 6205 2333
Website: www.cmsinc.org.au

Parents without Partners
This service can put single parents in touch with other single parents for companionship and support.
Tel: (02) 6248 6333
Tel: (02) 6258 4216 (after hours)
Website: www.pwp.freeyellow.com

Canberra One Parent Family Support
Provides advice and emotional support, a referral service, home visits, and assistance with housing, legal and financial issues.
Tel: (02) 6247 4282

NEW SOUTH WALES

Australian Breastfeeding Association (ABA)
The ABA provides a 24-hour help line for parents requiring assistance with breastfeeding issues. Educational information on breastfeeding is also available.
Tel: (02) 8853 4900
Helpline: (02) 8830 4999
Website: www.breastfeeding.asn.au

Australian Multiple Birth Association (AMBA)
The AMBA provides information and education, and counselling and support for mothers of multiple births.
Tel: (02) 9875 2404
Website: www.amba.org.au

Early Childhood Health Service
Look under 'Early Childhood Health Centre' or
'Community Health Centre' in the phone directory to
locate your nearest centre.

Leichhardt Women's Health Centre
Tel: (02) 9560 3011

Liverpool Women's Health Centre
Tel: (02) 9601 3555

Royal Hospital for Women
Barker Street
Randwick NSW 2031
Tel: (02) 9382 6111
Website: www.sesiahs.health.nsw.gov.au/rhw

Prince of Wales Hospital
Barker Street
Randwick NSW 2031
Tel: (02) 9382 2222
Website: www.sesiahs.health.nsw.gov.au/powh

Sydney Children's Hospital
High Street
Randwick NSW 2031
Tel: (02) 9382 1111
Website: www.sch.edu.au

Royal Alexandra Hospital for Children
Hawkesbury Road
Westmead NSW 2145
Tel: (02) 9845 0000
Website: www.chn.edu.au

Women's Information and Referral Service (WIRS)
Tel: 1800 817 227 (Free call)
Tel: 1800 673 304 (TTY)
Website: www.women.nsw.gov.au

Parent Line
Tel: 132 055 (9am-4.30pm, Mon-Sat)

Lifeline
Tel: 131 114
Website: www.lifeline.org.au

Relationships Australia, NSW
Relationships Australia is an organisation that offers
resources to couples, individuals and families to help
enhance and support relationships. By phoning the free
number below, your call will automatically be directed to
the nearest Relationships Australia office in your area.
Toll-free: 1300 364 277
Website: www.relationships.com.au

Family Crisis Service
Tel: (02) 9622 0313
Tel: (02) 9622 0522 (6pm–11pm, Mon–Fri; 10am–11pm
weekends and public holidays)

Karitane
Provides 24-hour phone advice for a variety of parenting
issues, also has a residential and day stay service.
Tel: (02) 9794 1852 (24-hour care line)
Free call: 1800 677 961 (STD callers)
Website: www.karitane.com.au

Tresillian Family Care Centres
Provides 24-hour phone advice for a variety of parenting
issues, also has a residential and day stay service.
Tel: (02) 9787 0800
Website: www.cs.nsw.gov.au/tresillian
24-hour Parents Help Line
Tel: (02) 9787 0855 (Sydney)
Tel: 1800 637 357 (country area free call)

Parents without Partners
This service can put single parents in touch with other
single parents for companionship and support.
Tel: (02) 9833 2633
Website: www.pwp-nsw.org

Single Parent Family Association
Tel: 1300 300 496

NORTHERN TERRITORY

Australian Breastfeeding Association (ABA)
The ABA provides a 24-hour help line for parents
requiring assistance with breastfeeding issues. Educational
information on breastfeeding is also available.
Tel: (08) 8411 0050
Website: www.breastfeeding.asn.au

NT Multiple Birth Club
Provides information and education, and counselling and support for mothers of multiple births.
Tel: (08) 8927 8968

Royal Darwin Hospital
Rockland Drive
Casuarina NT 0810
Tel: (08) 8922 8888

Alice Springs Hospital
Gap Road
Alice Springs NT 0870
Tel: (08) 8951 7777
Website: www.alicesprings.nt.gov.au/community/health_hospital.asp

Katherine Hospital
Gorge Road
Katherine NT 0850
Tel: (08) 8973 9211

Community Care Centres/Community Health Centres
Look under 'Territory Health Services' in the phone directory to locate your nearest community care/health centre.
Website: www.nt.gov.au/health

Women's Information Centre
The Women's Information Centre is a drop-in centre for women which offers free and confidential services. Additionally, they have an extensive referral and resource database for the Northern Territory area.
Tel: (08) 8951 5880
Website: www.womensinformationcentrealice.ths@nt.gov.au

Lifeline
Tel: 131 114
Website: www.lifeline.org.au

Parentline
Tel: 1300 301 300 (8am-10pm)
Website: www.parentline.com.au

Crisis Line
Tel: (08) 8981 9227
Free call: 1800 019 116

Relationships Australia, NT
Relationships Australia is an organisation that offers resources to couples, individuals and families to help enhance and support relationships. By phoning the free number below, your call will automatically be directed to the nearest Relationships Australia office in your area.
Toll-free: 1300 364 277
Website: www.relationships.com.au

QUEENSLAND

Australian Breastfeeding Association (ABA)
The ABA provides a 24-hour help line for parents requiring assistance with breastfeeding issues. Educational information on breastfeeding is also available.
Tel: (07) 3844 6488
BreastfeedingHelpline
Tel: (07) 3844 8166
Website: www.breastfeeding.asn.au

Australian Multiple Birth Association (AMBA) Qld Inc
The AMBA provides information and education, and counselling and support for mothers of multiple births. For your nearest contact, call the national office on:
Tel: (07) 3389 6382
Website: www.amba.org.au

Women's Health Queensland Wide Inc
Tel: (07) 3839 9962
Toll free: 1800 017 676
Health Information Line
Free call: 1800 017 676
website: www.womhealth.org.au

Royal Brisbane and Women's Hospital
Butterfield Street
Herston QLD 4006
Tel: (07) 3636 8111 (enquiries)
Website: www.health.qld.gov.au/rbwh

Royal Children's Hospital
Herston Road
Herston QLD 4006
Tel: (07) 3636 3777
Website: www.health.qld.gov.au/rch

Mater Children's Hospital Art Union
Free call: 1800 067 066
Website: www.materfoundation.com.au

Child and Youth Health
Look under 'Early Childhood Health Centre' or
'Community Health Centre' in the phone directory to
locate your nearest centre.

Women's Infolink
Tel: (07) 3224 2211
Free call: 1800 177 577
TTY: (07) 3321 3343
Website: www.qldwoman.qld.gov.au

Parentline
Tel: 1300 301 300
Website: www.parentline.com.au

Lifeline
Tel: 131 114
Website: www.lifeline.org.au

Relationships Australia, Qld
Relationships Australia is an organisation that offers
resources to couples, individuals and families to help
enhance and support relationships. By phoning the free
number below, your call will automatically be directed to
the nearest Relationships Australia office in your area.
Toll-free: 1300 364 277
Website: www.relationships.com.au

The Riverton Early Parenting Centre
Tel: (07) 3860 7111
Child Health Line
Tel: (07) 3862 2333 (24 hours)
Tel: 1800 177 279 (24 hours)

Brisbane Centre for Post-natal Disorders
Tel: (07) 3398 0238 (24 hours)

Parents without Partners Inc
This service can put single parents in touch with other
single parents for companionship and support.
Tel: (07) 3275 3290

SOUTH AUSTRALIA

Australian Breastfeeding Association (ABA)
The ABA provides a 24-hour help line for parents
requiring assistance with breastfeeding issues. Educational
information on breastfeeding is also available.
Tel: (08) 8411 0050
Tel: 1800 182 325 (country)
Website: www.breastfeeding.asn.au

Australian Multiple Birth Association (AMBA)
The AMBA provides information and education, and
counselling and support for mothers of multiple births.
SA Multiple Birth Association Inc
Tel: (08) 8364 0433
Website: www.samba.asn.au

Women's Health Statewide
Tel: (08) 8239 9600
Free call: 1800 182 098
Website: www.whs.sa.gov.au

Child and Youth Health
Look under 'Child and Youth Health' in the phone
directory to locate your nearest centre or contact:
Tel: (08) 8303 1500
Website: www.cyh.com

Women's and Children's Hospital
72 King William Road
North Adelaide SA 5006
Tel: (08) 8161 7000
Website: www.wch.sa.gov.au

Women's Information Service
Tel: (08) 8303 0590
Free call: 1800 188 158
Website: www.wis.sa.gov.au

Parents without Partners (SA) Inc
This service can put single parents in touch with other
single parents for companionship and support.
Tel: (08) 8359 1552
Website: www.sa.pwp.org.au

Parent Helpline
Tel: 1300 364 100 (cost of a local call)

Crisis Care
Tel: 131 611 (AH counselling from 4pm–9am, Mon–Fri,
24 hours over weekends and public holidays)

Lifeline
Tel: 131 114
Website: www.lifeline.org.au

Parenting SA
Tel: (08) 8303 1660
Website: www.parenting.sa.gov.au

Relationships Australia, SA
Relationships Australia is an organisation that offers
resources to couples, individuals and families to help
enhance and support relationships.
By phoning this free number below, your call will
automatically be directed to the nearest Relationships
Australia office in your area.
Toll-free: 1300 364 277
Website: www.relationships.com.au

Torrens House
Provides live-in programs for parents experiencing
difficulty with infants. Placement is by referral only.
Tel: 1300 733 606 (cost of a local call)
Website: www.cyh.com

Helen Mayo House
Helen Mayo House is an in-patient unit for women
suffering from a mental illness, including postnatal
depression
Tel: (08) 8303 1183 (24 hours)
Tel: (08) 8303 1425 (office number – 24 hours)
Free call: 1800 182 232

SPARK Resource Centre
This service provides parenting and education groups.
Tel: (08) 8226 2500

TASMANIA

Australian Breastfeeding Association (ABA)
Breastfeeding helpline and enquiries (South Hobart): (03)
6223 2609
For details of local contacts, see website:
www.breastfeeding.asn.au

Australian Multiple Birth Association (AMBA)
The AMBA provides information and education, and
counselling and support for mothers of multiple births.
Multiple Birth Association (southern Tasmania)
Tel: (03) 6272 0815
Website: www.amba.org.au

Hobart Women's Health Centre
Tel: (03) 6231 3212 (local)
Free call: 1800 353 212 (outside Hobart)
Website: www.hwhc.com.au

Family, Child & Youth Health Service
Look under 'Health and Human Services, Dept of' in the
phone directory to locate your nearest Family, Child &
Youth Health Service.

Royal Hobart Hospital
48 Liverpool Street
Hobart TAS 7000
Tel: (03) 6222 8308

Information and Referral Service
Women Tasmania
Tel: (03) 6233 2208
Free call: 1800 001 377
Website: www.women.tas.gov.au

Parenting Helpline
Tel: 1800 808 178 (24 hours)

Lifeline
Tel: 131 114
Website: www.lifeline.org.au

Relationships Australia, Tas
Relationships Australia is an organisation that offers
resources to couples, individuals and families to help
enhance and support relationships. By phoning the free
number below, your call will automatically be directed to
the nearest Relationships Australia office in your area.
Toll-free: 1300 364 277
Website: www.relationships.com.au

Lady Gowrie Family Support Service
Provides counselling, referrals and contacts for groups.
Tel: (03) 6230 6800

Lady Gowrie Tasmania Resource Service
Offers educational information and a library service.
Tel: (03) 6230 6800 (Hobart)
Tel: (03) 6443 5222 (Launceston)
Free call: 1800 675 416
Website: www.gowrie-tas.com.au

Parenting Centre
Tel: (03) 6233 2700

Walker House Parenting Centre
Tel: (03) 6326 6188

Parents without Partners Tasmania Inc
This service can put single parents in touch with other single parents for companionship and support.
Tel: (03) 6249 5215

VICTORIA

Australian Breastfeeding Association (ABA)
The ABA provides a 24-hour help line for parents requiring assistance with breastfeeding issues. Educational information on breastfeeding is also available.
Tel: (03) 9885 0653 (helpline)
Tel: (03) 9885 0855 (office)
Website: www.breastfeeding.asn.au

Australian Multiple Birth Association (AMBA)
The AMBA provides information and education, and counselling and support for mothers of multiple births.
Tel: (03) 9513 2050
Website: www.amba.org.au

Queen Victoria Women's Centre
The Queen Victoria Women's Centre has an extensive public library, which includes information about motherhood, parenting and child development.
Tel: (03) 8668 8100
Website: www.qvwc.org.au

Royal Women's Hospital
132 Grattan Street
Carlton VIC 3053
Tel: (03) 9344 2388
Website: www.rwh.org.au
Women's Health Information Centre
Tel: (03) 9344 2007
Free call: 1800 442 007

Website: www.rwh.org.au/wellwomens

Royal Children's Hospital
Flemington Road
Parkville VIC 3052
Tel: (03) 9345 5522
Website: www.rch.org.au

Maternal Child and Health Service
Look for Maternal Child and Health Services are under specific councils in your local phone directory, or to find details of local Maternal and Child Health Centres see:
www.office-for-children.vic.gov.au

Maternal and Child Health Line
Tel: 132 229 (24 hours)

Women's Information and Referral Exchange (WIRE)
Counsellors are available to give advice to callers on a wide variety of Women's issues, including parenting and family issues. Additionally, WIRE has an extensive referral database that can be used to assist callers to access appropriate services.
Tel: (03) 9921 0870
Telephone support: 1300 134 130 (9am-5pm, Mon–Fri)
Website: www.wire.org.au
Walk In Centre
Tel: (03) 9921 0878

Parentline
Tel: 132 289
Website: www.parentline.vic.gov.au

Lifeline
Tel: 131 114
Website: www.lifeline.org.au

Relationships Australia, Vic
Relationships Australia is an organisation that offers resources to couples, individuals and families to help enhance and support relationships. By phoning the free number below, your call will automatically be directed to the nearest Relationships Australia office in your area.
Toll-free: 1300 364 277
Website: www.relationships.com.au

Caroline Chisholm Society
The Caroline Chisholm Society can provide personal counselling, emergency accommodation and a number of

family support services to families experiencing difficulty. Material aid may also be provided.
Tel: (03) 9370 5122 (office)
Telephone support: (03) 9370 3933 (24 hours)
Free call: 1800 134 863 (24 hours)
Website: www.carolinechisholmsociety.com.au

O'Connell Family Centre (formerly Grey Sisters)

The O'Connell Centre is an Early Parenting Centre which provides support, education and assistance to families experiencing parenting difficulties with their babies and young children up to 4 years of age. The services offered include day stay programs, residential stay programs and education seminars, with the aim of assisting parents to feel more confident in parenting their children.
O'Connell Family Centre (Early Parenting Centre)
Tel: (03) 8416 7600
Website: www.mercy.com.au

Queen Elizabeth Centre (QEC)

The QEC is an Early Parenting Centre which provides support, education and assistance to families experiencing parenting difficulties with their babies and young children up to 4 years of age. The services offered include day stay programs, residential stay programs and education seminars, with the aim of assisting parents to feel more confident in parenting their children.
Tel: (03) 9549 2777
Website: www.qec.org.au

Tweddle Child + Family Health Service

Tweddle Child + Family Health Service is an Early Parenting Centre which provides support, education and assistance to families experiencing parenting difficulties with their babies and young children up to 4 years of age. The services offered include day stay programs, residential stay programs and education seminars, with the aim of assisting parents to feel more confident in parenting their children.
Tel: (03) 9689 1577
Website: www.tweddle.org.au

Council for Single Mothers and their Children Inc

This organisation provides single mothers with telephone support and information from other single mothers.
Tel: (03) 9654 0622 (9.30am–3pm, Mon–Thurs)
Toll free: 1800 077 374 (country callers)
Website: www.csmc.org.au

Parents Without Partners Vic Inc

This service can put single parents in touch with other single parents for companionship and support.
Tel: (03) 9852 1945
Website: www.pwp.freeyellow.com.au

Lady Gowrie Service

Offers children's services, educational information and a library service.
Tel: (03) 9347 6388
www.gowrie-melbourne.com.au

WESTERN AUSTRALIA

Australian Breastfeeding Association (ABA)

The ABA provides a 24-hour help line for parents requiring assistance with breastfeeding issues. Educational information on breastfeeding is also available.
Tel: (08) 9340 1200 (Breastfeeding Helpline)
Website: www.breastfeeding.asn.au

Australian Multiple Birth Association (AMBA) WA

The AMBA provides information and education, and counselling and support for mothers of multiple births. For your nearest contact, call the national office on:
Tel: (02) 9487 8825
Website: www.amba.org.au

Women's Health Service (Women's Health Care Association Inc)

Tel: (08) 9227 8122
Free call: 1800 998 399

Princess Margaret Hospital for Children

Roberts Road
Subiaco WA 6008
Tel: (08) 9340 8222 (enquiries)
Website: www.wchs.wa.gov.au

Child Health

Look under 'Child Health Centres' in the phone directory to locate your nearest centre.

Women's Information Service

Office for Women's Policy
Tel: (08) 6217 8230
Free call: 1800 199 174
Website: www.women.wa.gov.au

Parenting Line
Tel: (08) 9272 1466
Free call: 1800 654 432 (outside Perth metro area)

Family Helpline (24 hours service)
Tel: (08) 9223 1100
Free call: 1800 643 000 (outside Perth metro area)

Lifeline
Tel: 131 114
Website: www.lifeline.org.au

Relationships Australia, WA
Relationships Australia is an organisation that offers resources to couples, individuals and families to help enhance and support relationships. By phoning the free number below, your call will automatically be directed to the nearest Relationships Australia office in your area.
Toll-free: 1300 364 277
Website: www.relationships.com.au

Ngala Family Resource Centre
Tel: (08) 9368 9368 (8.30am–9pm)
Tel: 1800 111 546 (country callers)
Website: www.ngala.com.au

PND Support Association
Tel: (08) 9340 1622

Parents without Partners WA Inc
This service can put single parents in touch with other single parents for companionship and support.
Tel: (08) 9389 8350
Website: www.wa.pwp.org.au

NEW ZEALAND

The Plunket Service
National Office
Tel: (04) 471 0177
Website: www.plunket.org.nz

National Women's Hospital
Tel: (09) 307 4949
Website: www.adhb.govt.nz

USEFUL WEBSITES

There are many useful websites that provide information on the health and wellbeing of children and about parenting. We have included some websites as a starting point on your journey for more information; speak to your health professional as they can provide more information and details to you.

www.betterheatlh.vic.gov.au
www.raisingchildren.net.au
www.beststart.vic.gov.au
www.beyondblue.org.au